Handbook of Supervision:
A Cognitive Behavioral System

Dedication

To all the supervisors who have suffered through
Supervising with no clear guidelines
and
To all the supervisees who have suffered through
Supervision with no clear guidelines.

Handbook of Supervision: A Cognitive Behavioral System

William R. Leith, Ph.D.
Wayne State University
Detroit, Michigan

Elaine M. McNiece, Ed.D.
University of Central Arkansas
Conway, Arkansas

Betty B. Fusilier, M.A.
University of Central Arkansas
Conway, Arkansas

A College-Hill Publication
Little, Brown and Company
Boston/Toronto

College-Hill Press
A Division of
Little, Brown and Company (Inc.)
34 Beacon Street
Boston, Massachusetts 02108

Library of Congress Cataloging in Publication Data
Main entry under title:

Leith, William, 1927–
    Handbook of supervision : a cognitive behavioral system / William R. Leith, Elaine M. McNiece, Betty B. Fusilier.
        p.   cm.
    "A College-Hill publication."
    Bibliography.
    Includes index.
    1. Speech therapy—Study and teaching—Supervision.   2. Audiology—Study and teaching—Supervision.   3. Cognitive therapy.
I. McNiece, Elaine M., 1949–   . II. Fusilier, Betty B., 1943–   . III. Title.
RC428.L45   1989   88–23135
616.85′506—dc19   CIP

ISBN 0–316–52034–9

Printed in the United States of America

Contents

Acknowledgments

We wish to thank all those clinical supervisors who helped us develop and test the CBS system in various training programs around the country. Specifically we want to thank Kathy McDaniel, Kathy Roberts, Susan Moss, Robert Logan, Jim Thurman, and Jane Prince from the University of Central Arkansas, Beth Eaton and Terri Hutton from the University of Arkansas/Little Rock, and Kristine Sbaschnig, Kathy Williams, and Bill Wolfolk from Wayne State University. Not only did these people help us in field testing the system and make numerous suggestions to strengthen and improve it, they also participated as subjects in the reliability testing of the system.

We want to give special thanks to Dr. Eila Alahuhta and clinical supervisors Ritva Rauhala, Eero Suvilehto, Tarja Aaltonen, Anneli Ylihervo, and Orrokki Wilkman in the Department of Logopedics, University of Oulu, Oulu, Finland, for their early work in evaluating and testing the supervisory system on their undergraduate and graduate students in speech pathology. Their suggestions were invaluable as we developed the system.

We also want to thank Roe Scudder and the supervisors from the University of Wichita, Bob Shoewalter and the supervisors from Purdue University, and Brenda Antwine and the supervisors from Memphis State University for their invaluable comments and suggestions after testing the system.

Finally a special thanks to all those students who were supervised with the system during its developmental stages. And we all thank CVR for his major contributions to our field.

Preface

Perhaps the best way we can describe this book is to make clear what the book is *not*. This book is not a textbook in supervision, delving into the theoretical bases of supervision and reviewing and interpreting related research so that the reader can synthesize the information and establish his or her own philosophical approach to supervision. It also is not a book where the authors are setting forth their own general philosophical view of supervision and attempting to convince readers that this is the best way to view the process. Finally, it is not a learned, scholarly review of the literature in supervision to be used as a reference source. There are books written in the area of supervision that are representative of each of the above categories. We are not attempting to duplicate any other effort. Our book is concerned with a system of supervision, the theoretical base and the mechanics, if you will, of a behavioral view of the clinical process and a behavioral method of evaluating the clinician's performance in the process.

Anderson (1988) sets forth five stages in the supervisory process: understanding the process, planning, observing, analyzing and integrating. In this book, although we consider and discuss all stages of the supervisory process, we pay particular attention to the observational data-gathering stage. We chose to emphasize the observational aspect of supervision because we believe it is the weakest link in the supervision process. In order to gather data through observations, the first priority is that you know what you are looking for; you cannot make observations if it is not clear what you are observing. You must then know how to evaluate what you are observing. And in supervision, once they are evaluated, the data must yield some form of information that can be conveyed clearly and concisely to the person being observed. Our review of the literature in supervision demonstrated a desperate need for strengthening and standardizing the observational stage of supervision.

We do not take positions in the book regarding the frequency of supervision, the method used to share the information gathered with the clinician, whether the clinical conference is direct or indirect, whether the conference is supervisor-centered, clinician-centered, client-centered, or a combination of these views. These are matters best left in the hands of the supervisors themselves or the agency where the supervision is taking place.

The Cognitive Behavior Supervision (CBS) system presented here is unique in many ways, particularly in that it has an extensive theoretical foundation. The theoretical foundation is based on the concepts presented in Meichenbaum's cognitive behavior modification (1977) and is represented by the Clinical Interaction Model by Leith (1984). This behavior-oriented interactional approach to therapy is then the base of the Cognitive Behavior Supervision system.

In Section 1 of the book we present the clinical foundation of the CBS system. Chapter 1 presents an overview of supervision and its role in the training of a clinician. The theoretical basis of the CBS supervision system, cognitive behavior therapy, is presented in Chapter 2. In Chapter 3 we discuss the various roles that the supervisor and the supervised clinician play in various clinical settings where supervision occurs.

In the second section we present the CBS system in what we feel is enough detail so that it can be incorporated into any supervisory program for either the speech-language pathologist or the audiologist. Chapter 4 presents the Supervisory Clinical Interaction Model and its application in the supervisory process. The process of gathering data for evaluation is the topic of Chapter 5. Chapter 6 presents detailed operational definitions of the 43 clinical behaviors that the CBS system is designed to evaluate. Those clinical behaviors associated with the supervisor are then discussed in Chapter 7. Self-supervision, the goal of the supervision process, is the focus of Chapter 8. Chapter 9 consists of the operational guidelines for using the CBS system, including specific instructions on the use of the forms associated with the system. All forms, charts and scales associated with the CBS system are presented in the appendices.

There is no hidden agenda in this book. We studied the needs of the supervisor, the supervisee, and the clinical environments where supervision is provided, and then attempted to meet these needs. One of the main objectives of this venture was to develop a supervision system that removed some of the subjectivity from the process and that introduced some standardization to this important teaching function. We feel that the system we will introduce to you meets these objectives.

The Clinical Foundations of Supervision

Chapter 1

Clinical Supervision: An Overview

Clinical teaching, more commonly referred to as clinical supervision, is a crucial part of the training of the clinician. Much has been written about teaching styles and interpersonal relationships between the supervisor and the supervisee. Little has been written, however, about the methods the supervisor uses to gather data for her teaching, and even less about the criteria for judging the supervisee's performance of the clinical behaviors. This chapter deals with these issues and introduces clinical theory as a necessary foundation for any approach to clinical supervision. From this base, the advantages of the Cognitive Behavior Supervision (CBS) system are set forth.

PURPOSE OF THE BOOK

We are addressing this book to two groups of people. First, we have written the book for clinical supervisors, in both speech pathology and audiology, because we wanted to share with them a highly organized and objective supervisory system. The system is unique in many ways, but especially from the standpoint that it is based on a theoretical model of therapy. This theoretical foundation provides the supervisor with a reference point from which therapy can be viewed, a reference point that is then shared by all other supervisors using the same system. Further, this reference point is shared by the clinicians being supervised so there is a common point of view between supervisors and supervisees.

The book is also addressed to the clinicians, both speech pathologists and audiologists, who are in a training program where they are being supervised, be this as a beginning student in an academically-oriented training program or a professional clinician who is receiving specialized training in a service-oriented program to work with a unique clinical population. When we write about a "training program" we are talking about either programs that train students to become speech pathologists or audiologists, or clinical-service programs that train speech pathologists or audiologists to work in their special environment. The "supervisee," then, may be a seasoned professional or a new graduate working in a Clinical Fellowship Year (CFY) program.

We feel it is extremely important that the clinician being supervised has a broad understanding of the system being used to evaluate her. She should know specifically what clinical behaviors she is expected to perform. She also should know the criteria used in evaluating and grading the performances of each behavior. With this information, the clinician can feel more secure in her clinical interactions with her clients and her supervisor, because the "ground rules" for successful therapy are established and shared by her and her supervisor.

When the supervisor and the supervisee both have the same orientation to therapy and supervision, communication between them is enhanced. They will have the same theoretical foundations for their views of clinical interactions in therapy. They will use the same vocabulary to describe and discuss clinical experiences and observations. They will both understand the same clinical concepts concerning clinical interactions between the clinician and the client. We sometimes wonder how supervisors and supervisees communicate without this common base of knowledge and vocabulary. Perhaps this is the reason that some clinical supervisory conferences seem to resemble the architectural planning meetings for the Tower of Babel.

In a previous book, Leith (1984) presented the theoretical foundations of therapy, the laws and rules governing the teaching and learning interactions between the clinician and the client. These clinical interactions were presented in the form of a model, the Clinical Interaction Model (CIM). The CIM is basically a unique communications model that was designed to depict the rather complex interactions between clients and clinicians. With modification the CIM can be applied to all clinical/teaching interactions, including the complicated interactions between the supervisor and the supervisee. The model and its variations provide the clinician with a conceptual approach to these intricate interactions, which all professionals face on a daily basis.

Before getting much further into the book we need to identify the terms that will be used to identify people. For example, the *we* in the previous sentence refers solely to us, the authors, not to you and us as another form of "we." Now, the *you* in that sentence refers to you as a reader, while the *us* refers again to the authors, the *we* in the first sentence. If you have all of that straight, we can proceed. We will refer to all supervisors as *she*, because the majority of supervisors are female. We will also refer to all supervisees and clinicians as *she*, because again, most of them are females. However, so as not to be sexist in our approach, we will refer to all clients as *he*. Finally, because there are many more trainees in speech–language pathology than in audiology, which means there is more supervision in speech–language pathology, we have tended to emphasize the supervision of the speech–language pathologist in the book. We use the term *clinician* to refer to the speech–language pathologist for the sake of brevity and clarity. We trust that you, the language pathologist and the audiologist, will indulge us in our semantic folly and that, if you feel the need, you will substitute the word *language* or *audiologist* where you feel it is appropriate. We hope our plea for leniency is linguistically clear and does not fall on deaf ears.

DEFINING TERMS

Supervision

We must start out by attempting to define the term *supervision*. Perhaps, if we break it down into two words, "super" and "vision," it will give us some indication of what the term means. The word "super" means "extraordinary," or taking another view, it means "over something." The second word, "vision," is defined as "the act or power of sight or seeing." The first combination of definitions implies that supervision is "extra-ordinary sight." If this means hindsight, it is not too bad a definition of supervision since, at least in our experience, the supervisory conference considers mistakes that have already been made. If it means foresight, however, we are in trouble, since it would seem to suggest that we should foresee all of the clinical problems and avoid them. We have a feeling, just a passing feeling, that this perfect therapy is out of the range of most clinicians, and even supervisors.

The second combination of definitions, "extra-ordinary seeing," would seem to refer to someone who has exceptional eyesight. In thinking this over, a large number of the supervisors we have known wore eyeglasses. This would seem to exclude them from having exceptional eyesight. In fact, some of them do not even have exceptional insight or hindsight.

The third combination, "over sight," seems to refer to the clinical mistakes that clinicians make rather than being descriptive of supervision. In fact, "over sight" seems to be more the reason supervision is needed than a definition of it. Perhaps oversight is the justification for supervision.

Our last combination is "over seeing," and since it is our last combination it had better be a good one. Supervision, or better, clinical supervision, according to this definition would mean that the clinical interactions between the clinician and the client are being overseen by someone. We can then further imply that the person who is overseeing the clinical work is to be called a "clinical supervisor," and that he or she has expertise in the particular interaction. If there is no expertise, then the person is not overseeing but rather simply observing (which we will discuss shortly).

Good supervision is a skill that is learned over time. To dispel a common misunderstanding, supervision skill is not correlated with academic accomplishment. Just because a person has achieved a doctorate degree does not mean that he or she is a qualified supervisor. Such a person might be able to perform indirect supervision by acting as a resource and calling on his or her knowledge of the literature. However, in direct supervision, where the supervisor is evaluating clinical performance, the criterion for a good supervisor is experience as a clinician, regardless of degrees. One cannot evaluate and judge a process that one is not totally familiar with, regardless of the amount of information one has on the literature about any particular disorder. This means that the supervisor must be able to call upon her many years of experience as a clinician in her evaluation of clinical performances. It also means that the supervisor should have been an outstanding clinician during her clinical years. We do not mean to imply that all good clinicians automatically are good supervisors. As we said earlier, supervision is a skill that is learned. The supervisor must know what she is looking for when she observes therapy. She must have the tools to describe what is happening in therapy and communicate this and suggested changes in the clinical process to the clinician. She needs to be able to lead the clinician to the solution of the clinician's problems. Special training is necessary to learn these skills. Unfortunately, the amount and kind of training necessary to achieve this level of supervisory skill has yet to be determined. Much investigation is still needed in this area.

We cannot leave this discussion without considering the term *evaluation* as it relates to supervision. Evaluation is part of supervision. It is through the supervisory process that the supervisor is able to evaluate the clinical performance of the clinician she is supervising. This is the part of the supervisory process that yields the clinical "grade" for the clinician still in training. And it is this part of the supervisory process that is usually the most subjective and, in many cases, ambiguous. The supervisee wants to know what behaviors or actions she is being judged on and what the criteria are for grading. This is where most clinical supervision procedures break down, because there are no standard operational definitions of the clinical behaviors being observed and evaluated. Further, there are no specific criteria for grading performance, resulting in a process that is purely subjective; a nebulous creature with no limits, no boundaries, no laws, and no standards. This is the basis for the "free floating anxiety" (AKA hysteria) found in many clinicians involved in supervised clinical experiences.

The CBS system was developed to resolve this problem. It provides not only a complete list of operational definitions for all clinical behaviors that are to be evaluated, it also provides criteria for evaluation and grading, taking into account the level of clinical experience of the supervisee as well as how much "coaching" it took by the supervisor to get certain behaviors to occur. The system removes a great deal of subjectivity from supervision and it provides the supervisee with guidelines on how to operate effectively in the supervised environment. Yet, it remains flexible, adapting itself to any individual supervisory style and to an infinite variety of clinical settings.

Observation

We need also to consider the difference between supervision and observation. Although observation may be a part of supervision, supervision is not necessarily a part of observation. Anyone can observe something. All it takes is watching. There are observation ports in the barriers at many construction sites so that people can watch the construction. These people, fortunately, are only observing, not supervising the construction. Observation is a popular activity at beaches; men are observing women in their bathing suits who are at the same time observing men in their bathing suits. This is called observers observing observers. And we all recognize that there is no supervision involved in the observation of people at the beach. A lot of judgments and ratings perhaps ("Wow! There's a 10!"), but no supervision.

And, let us not forget that most of us started out in the profession by observing clinicians, usually other students about a year ahead of us, do therapy. We were deeply engrossed in observing the clinical interactions, wondering why the clinician was doing certain things and wondering how the clinician would react to specific things the client did in therapy. Little did we know that the clinician was wondering the same things at the time. Our clinical observations were a learning experience for us. They gave us some insight into what the profession was all about. But, we are certain you will agree, you were not in a position at that time to supervise the clinician.

The overseer or supervisor must have special knowledge and expertise in order to do the supervision. Therefore the supervisor is by definition an expert, knowledgeable in all aspects of the event he or she is supervising. And supervisor's observations are the basis for their "professional" appraisal of quality and quantity of the thing they are supervising.

Observation for clinical assessment is a unique form of observation. This invaluable clinical skill is not automatically acquired through clinical experience; it is a skill that must be carefully developed, as will be pointed out later in the book. But it is important to recognize early that observation is the most valuable means of data collection that the supervisor has.

Learning Experience: Hindsight, Insight, Foresight

How many times have you heard someone say that clinical supervision is a learning experience? Well, until there is a supervisory meeting between the clinician who did the therapy and the supervisor who observed the clinical interactions, the supervision is usually a learning experience only for the supervisor. She may never have seen therapy done that way before, and she may hope she never sees it done that way again.

Once there is a meeting between the supervisor and the clinician, the conference may be, but does not have to be, a learning experience. The type of interaction between the clinician and the supervisor will determine if learning takes place. The most basic ingredient needed in this interaction is good communication, which includes well-defined topics, a commonly understood vocabulary, commonly understood concepts, and an active interchange of knowledge between the supervisor and the clinician. If there is no good communication, learning is severely impaired.

We feel that the purpose of the clinical supervision meeting is for the supervisee to gain insight into her interactions with her client. She needs to know what she did wrong in the interaction and why it was wrong. She also needs to appreciate what she did correct and why her action was correct. The result of the conference should be that the clinician has a deeper and broader understanding of what transpired in the therapy session. And from this better understanding (insight) of the clinical interactions there should be better therapy planned for future clinical sessions and some foresight so that incorrect behaviors do not occur again.

Now, let's see if we can put this all together in a simple statement. If we failed to do this it would be an oversight on our part, or perhaps we would be shortsighted. So, we will say that clinical hindsight is the base of clinical insight, which in turn provides us with clinical foresight, which is the base of good therapy. Or, put another way, hindsight leads to insight, which gives us foresight. Why don't you stop here for a second and reread the last two sentences to make sure you have it.

Clinical Teaching

In this discussion of teaching, let us consider the clinician's role in therapy. We feel her purpose is to teach the client new speech or language behaviors, new concepts, new thoughts, and so forth. This is clinical teaching. So, the beginning clinician must learn various teaching methods to use with her clients. We assume she learns to teach by using modeling, giving the client guidance in behavioral performance, using rewards and penalties, or through the cognitive process by providing the client with information about a behavior performance, concept, or belief. However, we must then ask, who is teaching the new clinician how to teach? The first step in learning for the new clinician is observation; that is, watching another clinician doing therapy and then trying to imitate the model. Unfortunately, the clinician being observed is usually another student clinician who is just as confused as the observer. This is somewhat akin to trying to learn to swim by watching someone drown. Right or wrong, however, the foundations of the student's interactions in future therapy are established here. They must then be modified, shaped if you please, into a professional approach to therapy and clinical interaction. This, then, is the role of the supervisor, the "clinical teacher."

Clinical teaching is a term often used to imply that there are two distinct areas of teaching, one being apparently academic teaching and the other being clinical teaching. This is difficult to disagree with. Ask a variety of clinicians where they learned to do "therapy" and they will tell you they learned it, not in their regular academic courses in their training program, but in a special school; the school of hard knocks. They had to become involved in the interaction of therapy before they could learn the intricacies of the clinical process. And they needed to be guided through the process by an experienced clinician who would observe their therapy and discuss it with them. This person was their clinical supervisor, their "clinical teacher." And this teacher, as with all teachers, used various teaching methods, ranging from direct teaching in the form of a lecture which passed information to the clinician to indirect teaching in the form of discussions and providing references for the clinician to help resolve clinical problems. The former method seems more appropriate for beginning clinicians while the latter would be used with the advanced clinician.

Another way to look at clinical teaching is that the supervisor is primarily concerned with *how* the client is being taught while the academic teacher is more concerned with *what* the client is being taught. This is not to say that there is no overlap between the teachers, only that each has a particular focus. The supervisor's focus is on on-going therapy while the academic teacher is more concerned with providing information about a particular disorder so that the student can plan an appropriate treatment program.

Continuing this one step further, we note that most academic courses are "disorder-oriented," that is, they are concerned with presenting the student with information about a particular disorder. The student is presented with information concerning the etiology, behavioral descriptions, emotional aspects, and basic research into the disorder. On the other hand, clinical teaching, direct or indirect, is more comprehensive, more "process" oriented. It is not limited to a specific disorder but rather to the disorder as it relates to a particular client. And it involves discussions or "lectures," depending on the orientation of the supervisor, concerning interactional transactions, client motivation and attention, and teaching strategies. To put it more succinctly, academic teaching is more concerned with the theoretical aspects of disorders while clinical teaching is concerned with the pragmatics of therapy or treatment. Both areas of teaching must be present for the complete training of the clinician. And many supervisors incorporate both of these areas of teaching in their supervision.

Clinical Counseling

We include clinical counseling in our definition of terms since we believe it is part of the role of the supervisor. We are not talking about the supervisor providing counseling so that clinicians can resolve their personal conflicts. Rather, we are suggesting that the supervisor needs to recognize when a clinician's personal conflicts are interfering with the process of therapy. This could mean problems in interpersonal relationships with the clients, or with others involved in the process such as parents, other clinicians, or even the supervisor. The supervisor needs to be able to counsel the clinician so that she is able to recognize when her personal problems are interfering with therapy. The clinician must either extract her personal conflicts from the therapy interactions or be advised to seek professional help in eliminating the conflict.

SUPERVISION: A POINT OF VIEW

The Role of Clinical Theory

In Chapter 2 we will introduce you to a clinical theory that we feel clarifies the interactions between clinicians and clients, a point we consider essential for all persons involved in supervision of this clinical interaction. Let us address the question of why we feel it is important for you to assume a theoretical position for therapy. The principle is the same as the moral of the story of the six blind men attempting to describe an elephant. As the story goes, one man, standing at the side of the elephant, placed his hands again the elephant's side and proclaimed that an elephant was like a wall. A second man, crouching down feeling the elephant's leg, disagreed, saying that an elephant was like a tree trunk. Still another man was feeling the elephant's ear. He disagreed with both of the other men by stating that an elephant was like a big leaf on a tree. And so it went. The point is that all of the men were examining the same elephant, but each had a different frame of reference. Now, within limits, each man was correct in his description. Each had his own point of view, or "theory," and this provided him with a way of interpreting what he felt. In order to achieve agreement among the men there would have to be a single point of view or theory so they could all interpret their sensations the same way. The theory might suggest that the elephant had a number of different parts and that a systematic examination of all of the parts would be necessary before the complete picture of the elephant could be achieved. Even this most basic theory would result in a greater degree of agreement between the men.

In our example, however, each man was blind to the others' points of view. As we review the literature in the area of supervision, it reminds us of the time Tarzan (demonstrating a rather severe language disorder) said to Jane, "It real jungle there." Not only is there a real jungle out there, but there also seem to be a disproportionate number of elephants and blind men in the jungles of supervision.

Now, let us define *theory*. A theory is a systematic interpretation of an area, body of knowledge, or a phenomenon. Theory is important to you because, first, it provides you with a frame of reference, a means of approaching a phenomenon and understanding the information associated with it. Next, it provides you with a means of describing the phenomenon, a vocabulary directly related to the phenomenon.

Finally, it provides you with a means of interpreting or understanding your experiences with, or observations of, the phenomenon.

Our challenge is to introduce you, the supervisor and the supervisee, to a theoretical view of therapy so as to provide you with a frame of reference from which to view therapy, a vocabulary to describe your views, and a means of interpreting your clinical experiences and observations, both for yourself and to others. The main problem we will face in introducing our clinical theory will be one of semantics. Our clinical vocabulary is unique to our theory. We will introduce you to our vocabulary so that we may present our clinical theory in a clear and concise form. In case you are wondering, yes, we are dealing with another elephant.

Let us now apply this concept to clinical supervision. Without a basic theory concerning the interactions between the clinician and the client, each supervisor sees the interaction only from her own experiential background. Because no two supervisors ever have identical clinical backgrounds, and therefore have different points of view, there cannot help but be disagreement among supervisors, even though they are observing the same "elephant." This lack of agreement can have a decidedly negative effect on the clinician being supervised. She often cannot understand the supervisor's interpretation of her interactions with her client, because, again, her point of view differs from that of the supervisor. It ends up, in many instances, being a case of the blind leading the blind (pun intended).

The Statement of the Problem

We feel that there is a great need for a standardized supervision system. Such a system would eliminate the confusion we just described. This type of system is needed both by supervising programs and by the individual supervisor. The programs need the system so that all of the participating supervisors have the same orientation to supervision and are evaluating using the same criteria. In other words, they need such a system to improve the validity and reliability of their supervision programs. By also making all supervised clinicians familiar with the system, communication between supervisors and supervisees is improved. As a result, clinical teaching becomes more effective and efficient. There is also improved morale among the supervisees, because the subjectivity and abstractness of supervision have been reduced.

Let us consider an individual supervisor, a clinician who has just accepted a position as a supervisor in a training program. Unless she received her clinical training in that particular program, she will have to be introduced to the program's unique protocols and procedures for supervision. The problems she faces are:

1. What is the program's orientation to therapy? Is there any concern about interpersonal relations or is the concern focused on what data are presented to the client? Is there a standard clinical orientation or is each supervisor allowed his or her own unique interpretation?

2. How many forms are there and what specifically are they for? What are the procedures to use the forms?

3. What are the specific behaviors or other factors that she is to evaluate? How are the behaviors or factors described?

4. What criteria are used for grading? Is the grading adjusted according to the level of the clinician or are all clinicians, regardless of experience, graded on the same "curve?" Is the grading adjusted up or down according to the amount of supervision provided?

We are certain that there are other problems encountered when clinicians assume supervisory positions in training programs, but these are the major problems, or the major needs, if you will, of the supervisor.

There are, of course, programs where a supervisory system has been established

NOTES

for a long period of time and the protocols and procedures are documented so that new supervisory personnel can familiarize themselves with the process by reading about it. However, we feel that this is the exception rather than the rule. Due to time constraints and heavy supervision duties, many supervision programs do not have the necessary documentation to ensure continuity among new supervisory staff. It is a huge undertaking to write up an entire supervisory system; witness this book, our own effort. And if there is not a comprehensive documentation of the system, there is a resultant lack of continuity between the various supervisors in the program. Student clinicians are told one thing by one supervisor and another thing by another supervisor. And the students receive confusing evaluations because the supervisors are looking for different things and evaluating them by different criteria. There are serious problems with the validity and reliability of the supervisory system in many programs.

The Solution

The CBS system which we present in this book resolves these problems for both the supervision program and the individual supervisor. We feel it offers the following benefits:

1. It is based on a clinical theory and provides the supervisors with a common frame of reference from which to view therapy.
2. It sets forth the specific clinical behaviors that are to be evaluated and provides thorough operational definitions of all of the behaviors.
3. It provides a common clinical vocabulary that allows supervisor and supervisee to communicate effectively on a clinical concept level.
4. It provides a highly organized, systematic means of supervision in all areas of clinical functioning, yet is flexible enough to allow for individual supervisory "styles."
5. It allows for supervision of clinicians at all levels of experience, from beginning students to the practicing professional, providing differential criteria for rating clinical performance at the different experiential levels.
6. It can be used not only by the supervisor in the evaluation process but also by the supervisee in the development of her clinical problem solving, her self-supervision.
7. It allows for immediate feedback following observation or evaluation, as well as later feedback and discussion in the clinical conference.
8. It allows supervisees to know exactly where they are in the developmental process and what they need to do to improve.
9. It allows for behavioral goal setting at all phases of development.
10. It provides for relatively objective assessment and grading of clinical skills.
11. It is a complete system, well documented, providing all necessary supervisory forms, and is well tested in a variety of clinical environments.
12. It allows the supervisee to assess and provide feedback on the supervisory process to the supervisor, resulting in continued development and growth of supervisory skills.
13. It provides a means of supervision of speech, language and audiological practicum within the same system.
14. It is a reliable system, as demonstrated by the test-retest study reported in this book.

After much deliberation and systematic reviewing and comparing our many years of experience in supervision, we have included in the appendicies those laws of nature that influence all supervision, regardless of any attempts to eliminate or control them. We recommend you review these laws before reading further. These laws are found in Appendix A.

Chapter 2

Principles of Cognitive Behavior Therapy

Cognitive behavior modification provides the necessary theoretical base to explain clinical interactions between the clinician and the client. As such, it also forms the theoretical base for the CBS system. The learning orientation of cognitive behavior therapy is presented, as well as a glossary of terms used in discussing therapy. The theoretical base is then synthesized into a model form, the Clinical Interaction Model (CIM), which illustrates in detail the ongoing interactions in each clinical transaction. Methods of clinical planning and problem solving using the CIM are discussed. The special operant procedures of stimulus control, behavior shaping, and the token economy are then presented.

THE COGNITIVE BEHAVIORAL ORIENTATION

The discussion of cognitive behavior therapy that follows is in an abbreviated form. The unabridged presentation is contained in the book *Handbook of Clinical Methods in Communication Disorders* (Leith, 1984), and we recommend that, if possible, you review the material contained there for a more comprehensive understanding of the concepts involved in cognitive behavior therapy. Cognitive behavior therapy forms the theoretical base for the Cognitive Behavior Supervision (CBS) systems that is developed in this book.

As we discuss the clinical teaching and learning interactions between the clinician and the client we will approach them from both a cognitive and a behavioral point of view. Our approach uses concepts from both cognitive and "noncognitive" learning. It is important that we recognize the relationships between cognitive and noncognitive learning and that the client's cognitions, his thinking processes, are an integral part of both the development and the treatment of most communicative disorders.

In our discussions of the role of cognition in therapy, we will consider the cognitive involvement of both the client and the clinician. The client must perceive and comprehend the information presented to him by the clinician. The clinician must also be involved in therapy on a cognitive level; evaluating the client's responses, determining an appropriate response to the client's behavior, changing the clinical strategy if the client fails to respond or comprehend, and so forth.

Before we discuss theories and concepts of learning, let us clarify some of the special terminology we will be using. In operant conditioning, the terms *reinforce* and *punish* are often misunderstood. Because the terms *reward* and *penalty* are often used as synonyms for *reinforce* and *punish*, we will use them instead as we discuss operant procedures.

Also, when we apply a reward or a penalty we create different attitudes—different clinical cognitive sets—in our clients. With a reward, the client's attitude is positive and he performs those behaviors that yield more rewards. With a penalty, the client's attitude is negative in that he avoids performing the behavior that results in penalty. He will perform some other behavior so he will not be penalized. These different cognitive sets are very important, and we will be using both in our therapy. In order to identify them we will use the terms *Approach Motivation*, which is associated with rewards, and *Avoidance Motivation*, which is associated with penalty.

When a client's behavior is followed by something positive (reward), the client develops Approach Motivation. He is motivated to perform the behavior more often in order to get additional rewards. If the client's behavior is followed by something negative (penalty), he develops Avoidance Motivation. He is motivated to avoid the penalty by not performing the behavior.

We are now ready to discuss two of the more important learning concepts involved in cognitive behavior therapy.

LEARNING CONCEPTS

Cognitive behavior therapy uses concepts and principles primarily from two learning approaches, cognitive and behavioral. We will discuss each rather briefly and broadly. You should do some additional reading in learning theory for a broader and deeper understanding of the concepts presented here. We would recommend you read Lafrancois (1972) which is listed in the References and Recommended Readings section of the book.

Cognitive Learning

Cognition involves the perception of information, "thinking" about the information, and planning the response to the information. The aspects of cognition most important to the speech clinician are memory and problem solving. Also involved here is "observational learning," or learning through a modeling experience; it involves perception of the model, remembering the model, and then a cognitive involvement in attempts to imitate the model.

The two types of memory are long-term and short-term. Long-term memory implies that information is retained over long periods of time. In order for it to be retained, the information is rehearsed often, such as giving your name and telephone number or remembering information you received in one of your classes such as phonetics (you do remember how to read and write in phonetics, don't you?). The ability to remember information depends on how often you use it and recall it. If the information is not recalled periodically, it is "forgotten" (have you tried to make a phonetic transcription lately?). Short-term memory is for information to be retained briefly and then discarded. This allows us to look up a telephone number and remember it long enough to dial it, or to remember where we put a book down, or to remember the names of all the people at a party.

Now, where were we? Hummmmmmmmmm. Oh, yes! Both forms of memory are used in therapy. When we teach a new behavior or concept, we expect the client to remember it at least until the next therapy session. And, if we are going to be successful in therapy, the client must commit the new behavior or concept to long-term memory so it becomes part of his behavioral or knowledge system. If the client does not remember things from one therapy session to the next, each clinical session has to start from the beginning of therapy, each session being a new experience for the client.

Short-term memory is also important. We often give our clients instructions for performing a task or a behavior. If this information is not retained long enough to influence the performance of the task or behavior, we have a serious problem in providing therapy. If we present the client with a model of a behavior, he must remember the model long enough to see if he can imitate it.

Problem solving is extremely important in therapy, both in terms of resolving problems encountered in attempting to teach the client something and in planning the therapy program. This is the basis of self-supervision (which we will discuss in detail later). Problem solving is accomplished through insight. Insight is the sudden recognition of a solution to a problem. It is the light bulb that comes on above someone's head in a cartoon to indicate a sudden breakthrough. It is what happens when a person suddenly "gets" a joke. It is the sudden realization of the relationships between factors or bits of information. And this is a very common factor in our therapy; we model a behavior for a client and he must find a way to imitate it. We provide some information on, for example, how to produce an "easy vocal onset" and the client must then figure out how to do it. The client must integrate the information, see the interrelationships, and gain insight into the "problem" before he can produce the behavior correctly. You might give an articulation client the rules concerning phonology, which he must comprehend before he can apply them to his speech. He must see the relationships between the rules and his speech (gain "insight") before speech change can occur. Problem solving is important to both the clinician and the client.

Modeling a new behavior is perhaps the most common teaching technique used by the clinician. This is often referred to as observational learning. However, the clinician also uses auditory modeling in the form of presenting clients with the correct sound for them to imitate. It is important to recognize that this is a form of cognitive learning in that perception is involved, as well as thinking about how to imitate the model and evaluating how well the model was imitated.

Behavioral Learning

In operant or instrumental conditioning, learning depends on the consequence of the behavior; that is, what happens after the behavior is performed. If, according to the performer, the consequence is positive, the behavior has then been rewarded and the probability that it will occur again is increased. However, if the performer views the consequence as negative, there is a decreased probability of future occurrence of the behavior because it was penalized.

In this paradigm, we learn through rewards and penalties. If there is reward each time we perform a behavior, we quickly learn to perform the behavior to get the reward. However, if the consequence is a penalty, we stop performing the behavior in order to avoid the penalty.

Operant conditioning procedures are commonly used by clinicians, though not always correctly. Unfortunately, operant procedures appear to be quite simple and easy to apply. Nothing could be further from the truth. A simplistic approach to operant procedures actually does more clinical harm than good. One of the main problems faced in using operant procedures concerns the determination of rewards and penalties (but more about that later). Some therapy procedures are almost exclusively reward oriented, while others are mainly penalty oriented. But, in the main, most clinical applications of these principles are combined so that the client receives both rewards and penalties: correct speech behaviors are encouraged through rewards, while incorrect speech behaviors are discouraged through penalties.

ESTABLISHING A CLINICAL VOCABULARY

In order to discuss clinical interactions in therapy we need to establish a clinical vocabulary. The following terms will be used throughout the book as we discuss therapy and supervision.

NOTES

Behavior: A behavior is anything a person does. Overt behaviors are actions or movements that can be observed. Covert behaviors are thoughts or feelings that cannot be observed. There is a concept, known as the "dead man rule," which states that anything a living person can do that a dead man cannot do is considered a behavior. This should give us room to operate!

Behaviors have three characteristics with which we will be concerned; (1) their frequency of occurrence, (2) their strength or intensity when they occur, and (3) their duration once they do occur. We will be manipulating these characteristics as we move through therapy.

Stimulus (S): This is anything that attracts a person's attention. It may be something inside the person, such as a headache, or something in the external environment, such as objects in a room. We will not view a stimulus as an event that "elicits" a behavior, but rather as an event that prompts or cues a behavior to occur. The behavior may be either overt or covert.

Response (R): This is the reaction a person has to a stimulus. A response is a behavior. Responses include thinking about a stimulus, looking at an object in a room, imitating a speech behavior presented by the clinician, rewarding a client for a correct behavior, and other behaviors by either the client or the clinician.

Antecedent Event: This is any event that precedes a given response; that is, the stimulus that prompts or cues a response to occur.

Modeling: This is the demonstration of a behavior. We show the clients what we want them to do. Modeling could include such diverse behaviors as the production of the [r] sound, maintaining eye contact, opening the jaw further during speech, slowing down the rate of speech, using the correct syntax, and so on. This is the demonstration of the *behavior change goal* so that our clients know what we expect them to do.

Information: In our contact with the client we can either provide for the client, or request from the client, two types of information. First, we can provide *behavioral* information, which is concerned with the behavior we are attempting to teach. This type of information might include such things as telling the client to prolong the vowel when attempting to slow down the rate of speech, or to hold the teeth closer together when attempting to make the [s] sound. We can also request the client to repeat what we have said to him to make sure he understood us.

Second, we can provide *general* information. This might include a description of our therapy, therapy goals, or information to change attitudes or emotions. Again, we might ask the client to repeat what we have told him to determine his perception of what we said.

Guidance: Another term for guidance would be *prompt*. There are four types of guidance that we use in therapy. We give *verbal* guidance in the form of hints or cues about the performance of a behavior. *Gestural* guidance are those gestures we make to prompt or cue a behavior to occur. We also use *environmental* guidance when we manipulate the environment so that it elicits the behavior, such as showing the client a picture. Finally, we use *physical* guidance where we actually touch the client to assist in the performance of a behavior.

Contingent Event: This is any event that follows the response. Basically, this means either a pleasant event (reward) or an unpleasant event (penalty).

Reward (R+): This is the same as reinforcement. It signifies a positive event that occurs after a behavior is performed. If the event is truly rewarding to the client, the chances of the behavior occurring again are increased.

Penalty (P): This is the same as punishment. It signifies a negative event that occurs after a behavior is performed. If the event is truly penalizing to the client, the chances of the behavior occurring again are decreased.

Extinguish: When reward for a behavior is withheld, the behavior will extinguish. It will no longer occur since the reward is no longer presented and the behavior no longer has a purpose. However, if the behavior has become self rewarding it will continue to occur since it is no longer dependent on an external reward.

Reward Schedule: When we use this term we are referring to how often we reward a behavior. A *continuous* schedule means that we reward every occurrence of a behavior. This provides fast learning, but the behavior is not very stable and will have a tendency to be extinguished when the reward is removed. With an *intermittent* schedule we reward on a more random basis. There are two types of intermittent systems, *ratio* and *interval*. In the ratio system—either fixed or variable—the reward is given based on the number of times the behavior has occurred. In the interval system, the determining factor for reward is time. The intermittent schedule is not as efficient for learning a behavior, but makes the behavior very stable; the behavior will have a tendency to continue to occur even after the reward is removed.

Approach Motivation: This represents the mental attitude of the client when the focus of therapy is on rewards. He will perform the behavior being rewarded more often in order to get more rewards.

Avoidance Motivation: This represents the mental attitude of the client when the focus of therapy is on penalties. He will perform the behavior being penalized less often in order to avoid the penalty.

Shaping: This is the process of creating a *new* behavior in a client. As the client's behaviors more closely approximate the target behavior they are rewarded and through this process the new behavior is gradually "shaped."

Significant Others: These are people who are very important in the client's life. It may be the client's parents, foster parents, relative, wife, husband, or close friend.

Token Economy: This is when the client is initially rewarded with tokens, such as poker chips, which he can turn in at some later time for a more meaningful reward.

Stimulus Control: Stimuli can be manipulated or controlled in several ways. They can be gradually presented, gradually withdrawn, increased in number, decreased in number, or their prompting role changed.

Fading: This is the gradual removal of a stimulus. When we gradually withdraw the stimulus of our model of a behavior, we are fading the model. Also, when we gradually withdraw the rewards, we are fading them.

THE CLINICIAN–CLIENT INTERACTION

The clinical interaction between the clinician and the client is best viewed as a series of "transactions." We will discuss the transaction by using some of the terms we have just defined (see Figure 2-1). The interaction or transaction is initiated by the clinician providing a *stimulus* for the client. The stimulus may be a model of a behavior, a question asked of the client, or even information about a future clinical meeting. The clinician should have planned the stimulus according to her perception of the client's cognitive functional level. When the client, the *organism*, perceives the stimulus he thinks about it, deciding how to respond to the stimulus. When he does respond to the clinician, his *response* becomes the *stimulus* for the clinician. She, the *organism*, perceives the client's response and evaluates it. She checks the response for accuracy and frequency of occurrence. This information will tell her what her *response* will be, either a reward or penalty. She also evaluates the client's attending behavior. Only after making these judgments can she plan the next transaction. If all factors are satisfactory she proceeds to the next step in her therapy. However, if there is a problem with either the behavioral performance or the attending behavior of the client, she will have to make some corrections in the transaction and repeat the request for behavioral performance, or shift the focus of therapy to improving attending behaviors. She moves ahead in her therapy only when a transaction has been successful.

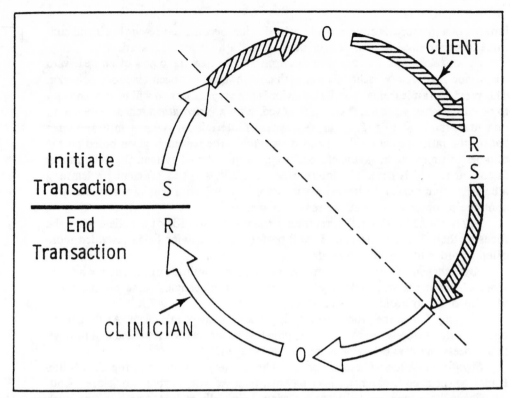

Figure 2-1. Clinical Transaction Diagram. The clinical transaction is initiated by the clinician's stimulus (S). The client thinks about the stimulus (O) and then responds (R). The client's response is the stimulus (S) for the clinician. She evaluates the client's stimulus (O) and then responds (R). This constitutes one clinical transaction. The clinician's next stimulus (S) initiates the next transaction.

NOTES

The clinician's response to the client is extremely important. If the response is a reward, the client will develop approach motivation. If the response is a penalty, the client will develop avoidance motivation. These forms of motivation are essential for successful therapy and are directly controlled by the clinician. Both motivational forms will be used in our therapy, so it is important that you recognize their basic differences. With approach motivation the client is actively seeking the reward, while with avoidance motivation the client is actively seeking to avoid the penalty.

There are *two* behavioral performances occurring simultaneously in each transaction; the *clinical behavior* that the client is performing and the client's *attending behavior*. Rewards and penalties will influence both forms of behavior. If attending behavior is rewarded, it will occur more often and, conversely, nonattending behavior will occur less often when it is penalized. If the client is not attending to therapy, the focus of the transaction may necessarily shift to dealing with attending behaviors.

Having completed the first transaction, the clinician initiates the second transaction. This sequence then continues, with the direction of each transaction dependent on the results of the preceding one. If you will, the transactions are like a string of beads, the clinician adding each bead to the string only after the preceding one is in place.

THE CLINICAL INTERACTION MODEL (CIM)

Clinical transactions, as shown in Figure 2-1, illustrate the interactions between the clinician and the client. It is a basic communications model and, as will become apparent later, can be applied to any number of clinical interactions, such as those between the clinician and a significant other and between the clinician and her supervisor. However, for now we will consider only the interactions between the clinician and the client. In all clinical interactions the clinician has three tasks she must perform in order for the transaction to be completed. Let us consider each of these tasks.

The Clinician's Stimulus (starting the transaction)

Modeling

As was stated before, modeling is perhaps the most common technique used by the speech clinician to teach a new behavior. We auditorily, and sometime visually, model sound productions. We model correct and incorrect productions so the client can identify each type. We model voice qualities. We model rate control for stutterers, and so forth. We are setting forth the correct behavior, the behavior-change goal, so the client can attempt to imitate it. Modeling is used as part of our clinical stimulus throughout our therapy. It is a tried and proven technique that gets positive results.

Guidance

This constitutes either directing the client to the correct behavior or prompting the behavior to occur. There are four types of guidance: verbal, gestural, environmental or physical. Verbal guidance is giving the client directions to improve his production of a behavior, such as saying to a client, "Don't blow so hard when you are making the [s] sound." Gestural guidance would consist of hand gestures or facial expressions that prompt or cue the client to perform a behavior or to modify it according to the gesture, such as gesturing to slow down for a stutterer who is attempting to speak at a new rate of speech. When the clinical environment is manipulated or changed to prompt a behavior to occur, that is environmental guidance. Placing a glass of water on the table to prompt the client to ask for it would be an an example of environmental guidance. This would also include removing distractions from the therapy room as a means of encouraging attending behavior. Physical guidance consists of directly assisting the client to perform a behavior. We might assist a stutterer in achieving relaxation by massaging the neck muscles, or increase the mouth opening in a voice case by pushing down on the chin during vocalization, or guide a client in the production of a sound by direct manipulation of the tongue position.

Information

First let us consider behavioral information. This is information we give the client about the behavior he is going to attempt to perform. We tell the articulation client working on the [l] to put the tongue up against the ridge behind the teeth, but to make the tongue narrow so it does not touch the sides of the mouth. On the other hand, general information is information we give to our client that is related to therapy, but not to specific behaviors. This would include making future appointments or giving him work to do at home.

We can also request information from the client, such as asking him if he understood what we just told him or asking him questions for a case history or a report. Periodic checks to see if the client understands what we are telling him or doing in therapy is a good way to determine if he is paying attention.

Most clinical stimuli consist of combinations of modeling, guidance and information. By varying the combinations the clinician can adjust the stimulus to the individual client. The stimulus can be made more or less complex, depending on the maturity and cognitive level of the client.

The Clinician's Cognitions

There are several very important decisions the clinician must make after the client responds. First, the correctness of the response must be determined. Second, any increase or decrease in the frequency of occurrence of the response must be noted. The clinician must also evaluate the client's attentiveness to therapy. Only then can she decide how she will start the next transaction.

The direction of the next transaction is determined by these three decisions. Depending on the correctness of the response she may move ahead in therapy or she may repeat the last transaction. If the behavior is not occurring more often she may have to adjust her reward/penalty system. She may also have to shift her therapy from focusing on the speech to dealing with the client's attending behaviors and his approach or avoidance motivation.

This is where the clinician does her problem solving, her self-supervision. It is here that she determines the effectiveness and efficiency of her treatment program. It is here that she makes adjustments and corrections in her therapy. She adjusts her therapy to meet the ever-changing needs, attitudes, emotions, and physical state of her client. She adjusts to shifts in the client's motivation, attitudes toward therapy, cooperation, and other factors that influence therapy.

The Clinician's Responses (ending the transaction)

Reward

If, following the behavior, an event occurs that the client views as something positive, it is a reward. The client is then motivated to get more of the reward by performing the rewarded behavior again. This is approach motivation and is extremely important to therapy. In selecting something that we will use for a reward, however, we cannot determine if it is truly a reward until we examine its effect on the client's behavior. It is only a reward if the client views it that way and the behavior occurs more often. We must check on the effects of our "rewards" in therapy, and if they are not increasing the frequency of occurrence of target behaviors, we must change them to something more appropriate for the client.

It is important to remember that the rewards we select are for our clients. Regardless of how much fun it is to dip into the client's candy rewards for a mid-therapy snack, this is a dangerous clinical behavior. Because it is rewarded by the candy, the frequency of dipping will increase, probably to the point where the client doesn't get any of the candy because the clinician has eaten all of it. This is especially true with chocolate candy.

We choose the client's rewards from two groups: primary rewards and secondary rewards. Primary rewards focus on basic needs, such as food and water. Secondary rewards are more social in nature and include such things as verbal praise or giving the client a token as a reward. Regardless of the type of reward, the strength, timing, appropriateness, and schedule of presentation of the reward must be considered.

The strength of the reward is related to its importance to the client. If the client highly values the reward, it is a strong reward. And, the stronger the reward, the greater the client's approach motivation. Keep in mind that the need or drive for a reward can be satiated. The first one hundred M&M's meet a need and are rewarding. The second hundred become a penalty. The relationship between the clinician and the client is also an important factor. If the client likes the clinician, the reward is more significant and stronger.

The timing of the presentation of the reward must be carefully attended to. If too much time is allowed to lapse between the performance of the behavior and the presentation of the reward, much of the effect of the reward is lost. The client must associate the presentation of the reward with the performance of the behavior. If the client performs the desired behavior and then scratches his nose and this is followed by the presentation of the reward, it is the scratching of the nose that is being rewarded, because the reward is contingent to that behavior.

The appropriateness of the reward relates to the clinical environment, the client, and other such factors. Food may not be an appropriate reward for the clinical environment. It may also present some problems associated with when the consumer consumes the food, because this could also consume a lot of valuable clinical time (a little play on words). Also, there is always the question of whether the parents will approve of candy or other sugar-laden rewards. Social rewards create fewer problems but may not have the strength you need to achieve high approach motivation. You will need to put a lot of thought into the selection of your rewards.

The two types of schedules of presentation of the rewards, continuous and intermittent, are very important factors for you to consider. In the continuous reward schedule, the reward is presented every time the behavior is successfully performed. Learning occurs very rapidly with this schedule but when the reward is removed, the new behavior fades rapidly. In order to combat the extinction of the behavior we shift to the intermittent reward schedule, in which we now no longer reward every behavioral performance, but more or less randomly present the reward for correct behaviors. Because the client is now waiting for the next reward, and cannot predict when it will occur, the effects of extinction are lessened. This type of schedule does not lend itself to rapid learning, but it does reduce the effect of extinction.

Penalty

Some therapy approaches depend heavily on the process of extinction; that is, if the incorrect speech behaviors are ignored and have no contingent event they will be extinguished and will no longer occur. The problem with this approach is that the incorrect speech behaviors are very strongly habituated and are self-rewarding in that they still accomplish their ends, communications and manipulation of the environment. In order to efficiently eliminate the incorrect speech behaviors, their occurrence should be penalized in some way. This could include saying to the client, "That was not very good," or, "I think you can do that better." This is negative feedback, a form of penalty. Penalty does not have to be harsh or severe. When the client interprets the contingent event as penalty, there will be a decrease in occurrence of the incorrect behavior, because the client wants to avoid the penalty. This is avoidance motivation.

As with rewards, we must verify that our response is being interpreted by the client as a penalty. We must also be concerned with the type of penalty we use. The two basic forms of penalty are by administration and by withdrawal. We can administer such penalties as requiring the client to repeat a behavior or giving him verbal disapproval. Penalty by withdrawal would constitute the removal of a reward, such as a token or a distracting object (for example, a toy car the client has brought with him to therapy). We can also remove the client from the clinical environment where he receives rewards, such as using the Time Out method.

The same general rules we applied to a reward also apply to a penalty. We must select a penalty that is appropriate not only for the client but also to the work environment. The strength of the penalty must also be carefully considered, as well as when and how often it is applied. As was stated earlier, the penalty need not be severe or harsh, just strong enough so that the client would prefer to avoid it. We must be careful to apply the penalty contingent to the inappropriate behavior and not to apply too much penalty, because this might have a negative effect on the morale of the client.

When we use penalty, we must be consistent in its application. Nothing is more disconcerting than to be penalized inconsistently for something.

There are people, including many clinicians, who object to the use of penalty with a client. However, their parents all used some form of penalty in raising them and they also use penalty in raising any children of their own. And if the clinicians are questioned closely, it becomes clear that they all use penalty in one form or another in their therapy. They just do not like to call it penalty. If we think carefully about all learning environments, penalty is a common feature. All societies use some form of penalty in maintaining social order; if there were no penalties in a society there would be no society, only anarchy. The penalty issue is also present in all classroom situations. Avoidance motivation runs rampant during examination periods. Avoidance motivation and penalty are valuable tools for learning in our lives, our society and our therapy.

The Model

When we combine the cognitive and behavioral learning orientations with the clinician/client transactions we form the Clinical Interaction Model (CIM) as presented in Figure 2-2. The CIM follows the basic [S - O - R/S - O - R] of the transaction, but is expanded to include the clinical behaviors of the clinician and client. It also shows the relationships between rewards or penalties, the client's approach or avoidance motivation, and attending behaviors.

The CIM is the basic model of all clinical interactions between the clinician and the client. With slight modification it is also applicable to her interactions with the significant others, the other professionals she deals with, and any other clinical contacts she makes. It also provides guidelines for planning therapy and for analyzing

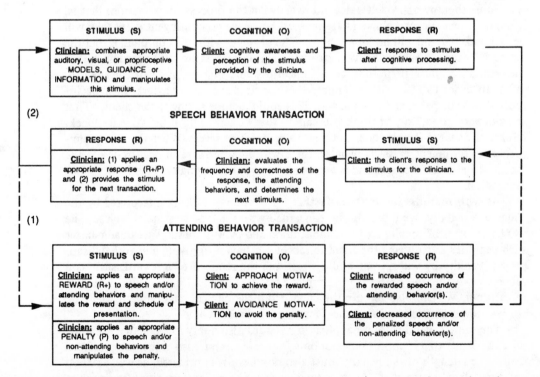

Figure 2-2. Clinical Interaction Model (CIM) illustrates the two clinical transactions that are occurring simultaneously in therapy. The clinician is attending to the speech behaviors of the client as well as his attending behaviors. The focal point of therapy is the speech behavior, but if the attending behavior becomes a problem, she can focus her therapy on the client's motivation and attending behaviors. Her response to the client, either reward or penalty, is very critical. It not only affects the occurrences of the client's speech behaviors, it also influences the client's motivation in therapy.

any clinical problems the clinician might have in therapy, such as the client not comprehending her stimulus or not attending to therapy.

The term *appropriate* is used in the CIM in conjunction with the clinician's stimulus and her response to the client. Appropriateness is a clinical judgment that only the clinician can make. The clinician's stimulus should be appropriate for the particular client. It should be tailored to his particular communication disorder, his age, cognitive functioning level, maturity, attitude toward therapy, and so forth. If the stimulus is not appropriate and the client does not learn efficiently from it, the stimulus will have to be modified, usually to a more complete stimulus or to a lower cognitive level for the client. For example, if the clinician presents the client with information that is beyond his cognitive level, constant repetition of the stimulus will accomplish nothing except to frustrate the client. For the client to comprehend the information the clinician must adjust it to match his cognitive level by rephrasing the information and/or changing the terminology used. If the clinician is requesting a behavioral performance that is beyond the client's ability, the client will again be frustrated. The stimulus and the goal behavior must be appropriate for the client.

The clinician's responses that provide rewards and penalties to the client must also be appropriate for the client in terms of what type of response is given and the way it is interpreted by him. The clinician must make an assumption of what type of response she feels would be appropriate and rewarding for, say, a seven-year-old boy. However, it is the boy's interpretation of that response that determines if it is appropriate and truly a reward. There are also rewards and penalties that are not appropriate for various clinical environments. The clinician must make this judgment as she assesses her work environment.

The CIM shows clearly the relationship between speech behaviors and attending behaviors. Appropriate rewards and penalties establish and maintain approach and avoidance motivation, which is the basis of attending behaviors. If there is no motivation, the client will not be attending to therapy. If this happens, the clinical focus must shift from the speech behavior to the attending behaviors. Learning cannot occur if the client is not paying attention. The clinician should, at this time, reevaluate the reward and penalty she is using and modify them if they have lost their effectiveness. With more effective rewards and penalties she could reward the client's attending behavior or penalize the nonattending behavior and, through approach and avoidance motivation, reestablish attending behaviors in the therapy process. Rewards and penalties should be reassessed periodically throughout therapy to determine their effectiveness. If either is no longer functioning according to its proposed clinical role, it should be changed.

As we conclude our discussion of the CIM we hope that you, the clinician, now see the CIM as a detailed communications model based on the theory of the cognitive behavioral approach to therapy. The laws and concepts that support the theoretical framework should now provide you with a point of view from which to view therapy. You should also have a vocabulary that explains events in therapy on a conceptual level rather than on an anecdotal level. The CIM will provide you a new means of planning therapy. And, in the event the teaching and learning interaction between you and your client is not effective or efficient, the CIM will provide you with a valuable means of resolving the clinical problem. The CIM will also serve you well in your self-evaluations, your self-supervision.

SPECIAL OPERANT CONCEPTS AND PROCEDURES

Stimulus Control

Our discussions of the stimulus thus far have been limited to the stimulus provided by the clinician in the CIM model. We will now broaden our view to include other forms of stimuli that influence the client. In general we will consider three types of stimuli: the people the client talks to, such as his parents and his teacher; the speaking situations the client encounters, such as reciting in class; and objects the client associates with speaking, such as the telephone.

When we use and manipulate these stimuli in order to prompt or cue a behavior to occur, this is stimulus control. This is very important in all phases of therapy, but it is especially important when we generalize the new speech behaviors to other environments. Our clients have become conditioned to respond in certain ways to various stimuli in their environments and these "conditioned" stimuli are a very important factor in our therapy. Let us first consider how a stimulus becomes conditioned.

Conditioned Stimuli

Stimuli are conditioned by consistently being associated with a reward or penalty, and once they are conditioned they "cue" the client as to what the outcome will be if a particular behavior is performed. Conditioned stimuli are referred to as *discriminative* stimuli. They do not *elicit* a behavioral response in a reflexive way, but rather prompt or cue the behavior to occur or to be avoided. Because the client knows what the outcome will be if he performs the behavior, he has some influence over whether or not the behavior occurs. Positive stimuli will encourage the performance of a response, because it will be rewarded. Negative stimuli will discourage the performance of a response so as to avoid the penalty. Thus, conditioned stimuli have a direct influence on the probability of the behavior occurring.

POSITIVE STIMULI. These are stimuli that have been conditioned to a positive outcome, a reward. They are designated by S+. A dip in a pool on a hot day has become an S+ to most of us. The pool symbolically implies that if we jump in, the outcome will be rewarding. The pool was not always a conditioned stimulus. It became a conditioned S+ only after we had jumped in on a hot day and found it rewarding. An association was then made between the pool and the reward of being in it.

Stimuli in the therapeutic environment can quickly assume the role of S+. When the clinician rewards speech behavior, she is associated with the reward and becomes an S+. So, her very presence cues the client that if he performs the specific speech behavior, he will be rewarded. The entire clinical environment becomes an S+, cueing the rewarded behavior to occur. When there is no S+ to prompt the new speech behavior to occur, the incorrect behavior occurs. This explains why carry-over is so difficult to achieve unless significant others have been involved in therapy and have assumed an S+ role.

NEGATIVE STIMULI. Stimuli that are associated with a negative outcome, a penalty, become a negative stimuli or S−. These cues, for example, influence the way we drive our cars. Consider speed limits that are posted on highways. A large number of drivers exceed this speed, that is until a police car, an S−, is sighted. Traffic suddenly assumes the posted speed limit so as to avoid receiving a speeding ticket, a rather severe penalty. These drivers know they are breaking the law, so while the police car is visible, they do not perform the illegal behavior of speeding in order to avoid the ticket. But, the minute the police car is out of sight, back to the speeding. This must be the basis for the adage, "Out of sight, out of mind." Signs also serve as S− cues telling you to avoid something: "Do Not Enter," "No Left Turn," "Beware of the Dog," and (depending on your sex) "Men."

If the clinician consistently penalizes an incorrect behavior, she assumes the role of S− for that behavior. The behavior may be disruptive, such as wandering around the clinic room, nonattending behavior in the form of looking out the window, or an incorrect speech behavior. The S− role is important, not only in direct therapy, but also in establishing control over clients whose general behaviors interfere with therapy.

The effects of penalty are complex. They do not extinguish a behavior, only reduce its frequency of occurrence to a very low point. If the application of penalty is excessive, it could lead to loss of motivation, fear, tension or anxiety. This does not mean that we do not use penalty in our therapy, only that we must understand what the ramifications are and apply penalty accordingly.

NEUTRAL STIMULI. In addition to the stimulus roles of S+, prompting the correct production of the speech behavior, and S−, prompting the avoidance of the penalty by not producing the incorrect behavior, the stimulus can assume a third role, a neutral stimuli or S0. This stimulus cues that there will be no consequence for the behavior. And if there is no reward, the behavior has no purpose and ceases to occur. Behaviors are extinguished by removing all rewards.

Stimulus Manipulation

These conditioned stimuli can be manipulated in a number of ways and this is very important to our therapy. The five forms of stimulus manipulation are discussed below.

SHIFTING THE ROLE OF THE STIMULI. Although a stimulus may have been conditioned to an S+, S−, or S0 role, these roles can be changed. We change the stimulus role by associating the stimulus with a different contingent event. If the parents penalized the client for his voice quality, their role is an S−. However, if they are counseled so that they no longer react to the voice, their role will shift to S0. If a significant other rewards an incorrect speech behavior, they are an S+, maintaining that behavior. Their S+ role can be shifted to an S0 by removing the reward. This shifting is an important factor when we establish a home program or when we generalize the new speech behavior to environments outside the clinic room.

GRADUAL INTRODUCTION OF STIMULI. If an S− is too threatening and overwhelms the client, we may find that we must introduce the S− gradually, allowing the client time to adjust to it. A client who stutters may find it extremely frightening to speak in front of a group. When he is in front of a group, he is so frightened that he cannot use his new speech behaviors. We can gradually introduce this S− situation by starting with one listener. When the client can perform satisfactorily with one listener and the situation becomes an S+, we can then add another listener. This process is repeated. In this way we gradually introduce the stimuli while keeping the situation at an emotional level where the client can perform his new speech behavior. The speaking situation gradually then shifts from an S− to an S+ (or at least to a very weak S−) as he learns that he can speak in front of a group. In this example we are gradually increasing the strength or intensity of the stimulus. We can also manipulate the frequency and the duration of stimuli if and when the need arises.

GRADUAL WITHDRAWAL OF STIMULI. The stimulus can also be gradually withdrawn or faded. We do this by presenting it less often (frequency), in a weaker form (strength or intensity), or for a shorter period of time (duration). We can fade the stimulus as the client learns the new speech behavior or we can fade the influence of our S+ role by not rewarding as much. Fading makes the new speech behavior more independent. We must eventually fade all stimuli so that the new speech behavior is being performed independent of prompts or cues. When this is happening, we can terminate therapy.

INCREASE THE NUMBER OF STIMULI. We must increase the number of S+ in the client's speaking environments in order to achieve carry-over of the new speech behavior. These S+ will cue the new speech behavior to occur in other environments, such as in the school, the home, on the job. This form of manipulation is dependent on the client's significant others or cooperative people in the environments. This form of stimulus manipulation is extremely important. The efficiency of our therapy in terms of generalizing the new speech to other speaking environments is dependent upon the number of S+ in the client's life.

DECREASE THE NUMBER OF STIMULI. We may also find the need to reduce the number of stimuli in the client's clinical environment. The stuttering client may be overwhelmed by the number of other clients in a group or other distractions in the clinical room. If the client cannot function in a large group, he might be placed in a smaller group or even given individual therapy until he can handle a small group (gradual introduction of stimuli). If a client is distracted by objects in the clinic room, perhaps some of them can be removed.

Procedures for Delivery of Rewards and Penalties

There are two special operant procedures that can be used to present rewards and penalties. Shaping is concerned with what behavior is rewarded, while the token economy concerns what is used as a reward. The procedures are not mutually exclusive; they may be combined into a token economy using the shaping procedure.

Shaping

When the clinical task is to create new behaviors in the client, shaping is used. In its purest form, this procedure does not identify the goal behavior for the client. The behaviors that do occur in this process are not goal oriented but, rather, more or less random in nature. Behaviors that approach the goal behavior are rewarded, while all other behaviors are ignored. The reward increases the probability that goal-oriented behaviors will occur again. Behaviors that are not rewarded are extinguished. The criterion for reward is gradually changed to focus on the goal behavior so that eventually this is the only behavior that will be rewarded. This process is known as "successive approximation."

When the speech clinician uses the shaping technique, she improves the efficiency of the process by providing the client with the goal behavior through modeling, guidance, and information. Since the client then knows the goal behavior, all of his behavioral attempts are goal oriented. The process is also supplemented by including cognitive learning through guidance and information she provides for the client. It is important that the clinician recognize that human learning occurs in gradual steps, not all at once.

Token Economy

The token economy is a procedure for administering rewards (or penalties) to a client. Two problems encountered when giving a specific reward to a client are that (1) the client may become bored or satiated with the reward and (2) in a group situation it is almost impossible to find a single reward that is appropriate for all group members. The token economy solves both of these problems.

Tokens can be anything identified by the clinician as having "purchasing power," for example a poker chip. Clients get tokens as rewards during therapy time and then redeem them for a tangible reward, a "backup reward," at the end of therapy or at another designated time. When the client realizes that the tokens have purchasing power, the tokens themselves become rewarding.

The token economy allows the clinician freedom to select a variety of items as backup rewards. With a variety of rewards, each client can choose the reward he wants. The clinician can also set "prices" for the rewards. If a client wants an "expensive" reward, he will have greater approach motivation to get tokens so he can purchase the item.

Penalty can also be included in the token economy, losing a token if a behavior is performed incorrectly. The clinician can use this form of penalty to create avoidance motivation. The client will avoid performing the incorrect behavior to prevent the clinician from removing a token. The clinician is now creating both approach and avoidance motivation in the client. This will be a very effective and efficient therapy.

Some advantages of token rewards over traditional rewards are providing a variety of rewards, not needing to interrupt therapy while the client "consumes" a reward, making it easier to administer the reward, and giving the same initial reward to all clients in a group setting. The token economy is an extremely useful clinical tool for the speech clinician.

As we conclude our presentation of cognitive behavior therapy we again stress that the practical clinical application of these principles, as presented in the CIM, should form the core of your therapy. We also suggest that the effectiveness and efficiency of your therapy will be enhanced, particularly in the later phases, through the use of the principles set forth in the section on stimulus control. And finally we would urge you to include the techniques of shaping and the token economy in your clinical repertoire.

Chapter 3

Clinical Roles in Supervision

There are many roles played both by the supervisor and the supervisee in their interactions in the supervision process. These roles are first discussed under the heading of "games" played by both parties involved in the interaction. The discussion then focuses on the supervisor's roles as defined by her place of employment. The final part of the chapter deals with the roles of the supervisee as defined by her status as a student, a professional receiving special training and as a professional providing herself with self-supervision.

INTRODUCTION

Thus far we have presented an overview of supervision and an introduction to cognitive behavior therapy that provides the theoretical foundation of that therapy. We now need to consider the various roles assumed in supervision by the supervisor and the supervisee. Although the supervisor always assumes the role of "teacher" and the supervisee is always in the role of "student," there are, depending on the clinical environment where the supervision takes place, many variations in the roles. The roles constitute the clinical interaction between the supervisor and the supervisee, and nowhere is this interaction more apparent and more crucial than in the clinical conference. Sometimes the supervisory roles and the clinical interaction are overshadowed and even replaced in the conference by personal needs which are manifested in nonclinical roles played by either the supervisee or the supervisor. These nonclinical roles played in the conference result in interpersonal "games," which interrupt the teaching activities of the conference. Although we are not directly concerned with the interpersonal games that may or may not be played out between the supervisor and supervisee, Sleight (1984), in a very cogent and humorous discussion of the topic, lists four categories of games played by the supervisee; Manipulating Demand Levels, Redefining Relationships, Reducing Power Disparities, and Controlling Conferences. For the supervisor, she lists only one category; Supervisor-initiated Games. In that these clinical conference games so directly influence the conference roles of the supervisor and the supervisee, we will review them and introduce some of our own interpretations.

GAMES PLAYED IN SUPERVISION

In the category of Manipulating Demand Levels, Sleight lists the game "See People, Not Plans." Actually, as Sleight points out, this game is played by both the supervisor and the supervisee. It has to do with reactions to written work, and how both the supervisor and the supervisee are, at times, overwhelmed with paper work.

As anyone knows who has been a supervisor or been supervised, the reports, evaluations, reevaluations, evaluations of the reevaluations, reports on the reports, evaluations of the reports on the reports and so forth become very tedious at times. So, the theme of the game is, "Let's all deal with the clients and forget all the written work." At first glance this looks like a good idea, but what would everyone involved do with the time released from the paper work? With too much time on their hands they would probably just get into trouble.

The next game is "Be Nice to Me Because I Am Nice to You." The theme in this game is, "Flattery will get you everywhere!" All the supervisee has to do is establish the tone of the conference by telling the supervisor what a brilliant person she is, or how stylish she dresses, or how nice her hair looks. From this point on the supervisor will think twice about making some unflattering comment about the supervisee's therapy.

Category two, Redefining Relationships, starts with the game "Poor Me." Now, obviously, this sympathy game could also be played by all supervisors, but it is the supervisee's game. Once the supervisee starts by sharing her problems (grades, tests, the family, finances, boyfriends, and so forth) with the supervisor, it is very difficult for the supervisor to refocus the conference on mundane matters such as the supervisee's performance in therapy. Maybe the way around this is for the supervisor to tell the supervisee her problems, which of course would be bigger and better; the first liar won't have a chance.

The next game is "Evaluation Is Not for Friends." If the supervisee can establish a friendship with the supervisor, the critical evaluation of clinical performance is softened. Who can be that hard on a friend? Beware of supervisees bearing gifts!

Reducing Power Disparities is the next category. It is obvious that the power rests with the supervisor. But all supervisees are survivors. All they have to do is establish their own power base and they are secure. The first game is "Have You Read This Month's *JSHD* Yet?" This is what is referred to on the street as "dirty pool." If the supervisor says she has read it, the supervisee, who has reviewed the journal just before the conference, asks about very specific and minute bits of information. Sooner or later she has the supervisor trapped. This game is part of a bigger game called "gotcha."

In the game "So What Do You Know About It" the supervisee finds some clinical experience she has had that the supervisor has not had. Once she finds this experience she can refer to it whenever she feels the conference is getting out of hand. This is also a game of "One-upmanship." She can always put the supervisor "in her place" by referring to her "limited" experiences.

And then there is the lowest blow of all, the most vicious game, "But The Doctor Says...." This game does not work well with supervisors who have the doctorate, but it really establishes a balance of power with the supervisor who has the master's degree. When confronted with a supervisor who has the doctorate, the supervisee then refers to the Doctor who teaches the course in the particular disorder they are discussing. This game might also be called the "Mexican Standoff."

In the category Controlling Conferences, the games are designed to determine who is in charge of the clinical conference. The first game, "I Have a Little List," concerns a lengthy list of questions the supervisee has written down to ask the supervisor. Obviously, answering all the questions occupies most of the clinical conference and there is just not enough time to get to the real business, the supervisee's performance in therapy. If the supervisee spent as much time preparing her therapy as she spent making up the list, the conference would probably have been the best either of them ever had. One can only hope that the questions are good ones and that the supervisee learns something from the conference. We also hope the supervisor learns something from this experience: to be on the lookout for this game in the future.

The really slick game in this category is called "Head Them Off at the Pass." In this game the supervisee arrives at the conference with her own lengthy list of problems she is having with her therapy. And the longer she makes her list, the less the supervisor gets to say. Now, how could the supervisor help but feel some sympathy for the supervisee who comes in with a list of 72 problems she experienced in one therapy session, some of which are obviously not even problems. Any humane supervisor would have to try to make the supervisee feel better about her performance, especially pointing out those items on the list that are really not problems. Gotcha!

In the "Little Old Me" game, the supervisee turns to the supervisor for all clinical guidance with her client. She indicates that the clinical problem is beyond her capabilities. So, she turns the client over to the supervisor whose great wisdom and clinical skill will save the poor soul from a fate worse than death. And if the supervisor takes the bait—Gotcha!

Every supervisor who has supervised for more than a week has been involved in the next game, "But Ms. Smith Liked It That Way." "Who is Ms. Smith?" you ask. She was the supervisor the supervisee had last semester. So now we have another Mexican standoff. We might even call this game, "Will The Real Expert Please Stand?"

The last game in this category is "Losing My Cool." The clue that this game is about to be played is when the supervisee arrives for the conference either armed with a box of tissues or comes storming into the conference ready to do battle. The theme to the first approach is, "You're going to make me cry," a rather common theme in conferences, while the theme for the second approach is, "The best defense is a good offense." In either approach, the supervisor is put into a defensive mode, having to deal with the supervisee's emotions rather than the issue of clinical performance. This game is enough to make a supervisor cry.

Now, there are also some games that the supervisor plays, and Sleight lists two. The first game is "I Wonder Why You Said That?" This is the game supervisors play when asked a question by the supervisee that they cannot answer. This seems to imply that there is a three word phrase, somewhat like a four letter word, that supervisor's cannot not utter, that being, "I don't know." The ploy here is to shift the focus, to suggest that the supervisee is playing a game; accuse before being accused.

The second game is "One Good Question Deserves Another." Always answer a question by asking a question. Does this sound a lot like the first game? The supervisee says, "Should I use the Zyykeptij approach with Mr. Smith?" And the supervisor then says, "Well, what do you think about this?" This may be a coverup for a lack of information about this particular approach or it may be a ploy on the part of the supervisor to encourage problem solving on the part of the supervisee. In this case our bet is on the former rather than the latter purpose, that the supervisor does not know what the Zyykeptij approach is. Come to think of it, neither do we.

These are the only two games that Sleight lists for the supervisor. We would like to suggest some others and let you, the supervisees, decide from the name of the game what the theme of the game is. You may also add to our list, but we would ask you to limit yourself to 35 games. We suggest the following games:

Is This a Waste of Time or What
You Are at the Shrine
Supervisees Are to Be Seen, not Heard
Catch'm Off Guard
Wheel of Misfortune
Off with Her Head

Now that we understand the dynamics of the clinical conference, let us consider the various roles that the supervisor and the supervisee must play in a variety of clinical settings.

VARIATIONS IN THE ROLE OF THE SUPERVISOR

In the Training Program

It is impossible to set forth a specific role for supervisors in a training program, because there is a great deal of variation in duties and responsibilities among programs. However, we will discuss the variations of this role as we see them. There is no problem with the relationship the supervisor has with the student clinician; she is indeed the clinical teacher. The problem that may arise concerns what constitutes her areas of teaching. As we consider who should teach the academic information—the anatomy, physiology, etiology and research findings associated with specific disorder types—we feel, without much fear of dissension, that it is the proper role of the academic faculty member who teaches the course or courses associated with the specific disorder. However, there is a gray area constituted by the teaching of the diagnostic and therapeutic procedures to be used with the disorder. We now have the grounds for conflict. There are several variations to this. One view is that if the academic faculty member includes diagnostic and therapy procedures in the academic course on the disorder, the supervisor has a moral, if not ethical, obligation to follow the academic faculty member's procedures and assist the student clinician as she learns to perform the procedures. It would seem a bit presumptuous for a supervisor to overrule the academic faculty member, discounting the course material as irrelevant, and attempting to teach the clinician an entirely new diagnostic and therapeutic approach to the disorder. The academic faculty member has spent years in studying the disorder and is, in every sense of the word, an expert in this disorder. And as the individual who taught the clinicians about the disorder, his diagnostic and clinical approach should be honored. If the supervisor is not familiar with the approach, it is her obligation to learn it, because she is supervising in the program where the faculty member is a teacher.

The second view here is that the supervisor has been trained in a certain way to approach a specific disorder and, in order to teach the student clinician a diagnostic and clinical approach, she must teach the one that she understands and has used. Therefore, when she is assigned to supervise the treatment of a specific disorder, she teaches the clinician her approach and has it applied in therapy rather than the approach taught in the classroom. Teaching a complete approach to a disorder type within the time limits imposed in a supervision schedule is a massive undertaking. The student may have the necessary background information on the disorder type, but the new approach to diagnostics and treatment constitutes a major teaching task, because it involves reinterpretation of the etiology of the disorder as well as the research findings associated with the behavioral phenomenology of the disorder. There will of necessity be a lot of confusion as the student attempts to comprehend the supervisor's clinical approach while viewing the disorder from the point of view expressed in the classroom. It might be simpler and more time-effective for the experienced and knowledgeable supervisor to learn the approach taught in the classroom.

There is a third possibility, which is not as common as the others, or as popular with many academic teaching faculty, where all teaching faculty are also expected to supervise. When possible, clients are assigned for supervision according to the specialty of the faculty member. But, regardless of what type of client is assigned to which supervisor, the assigned supervisor is considered the expert in the treatment of the disorder. This discourages the game "But the Doctor Says...." This arrangement may increase the communication between the teaching faculty and the supervision faculty, but it could also create some very delicate situations in terms of the individual supervisor being the "expert" in another faculty member's area of specialty. This would be especially true if the faculty member strongly advocates one side of the clinical treatment coin and the supervisor advocates the other.

All of these approaches to supervision create some problems, not only in the academic environment but also in the agency environment where a specific clinical approach is used, as will be discussed later. The problem cannot be avoided, because the supervisor is expected to supervise all disorder types and to be an expert with all of them, and no one can be an expert in all disorders. There are no easy answers to these role problems. Each supervisor needs to assess her own working environment and take the approach that is appropriate for the training program.

There is a fourth possibility here, one that resolves all the supervision problems but that certainly introduces other problems we do not have space to deal with here. This is where the academic faculty members do not get involved in diagnostic and therapeutic procedures. This allows the supervisor freedom to approach the diagnosis and treatment of the disorder type without fear of conflict with a faculty member. The clinicians also benefit from this arrangement, because competing, and often conflicting, information is not presented.

We feel that the conflict between academic faculty and clinical supervisors most often occurs with disorder types having more theoretical etiology and treatment programs, such as language disorders and stuttering. With these disorder types it is more likely that the faculty member teaching the course will take a theoretical stand and teach diagnostics and therapy based on the theoretical position. Having taken a professional position, the faculty member will view any clinical variation from the clinical approach taught in the classroom as heresy, as a personal challenge to his or her professional qualifications with the disorder. If the instructor in these disorder courses assumes no theoretical position but rather teaches other's theories and therapies, there is no emotional involvement, no professional commitment, and no conflict with the supervisor who teaches her own approaches. With disorder types where there is no controversy among experts on the etiological or theoretical bases, there is a minimum of conflict, because the faculty member is not taking a firm stand on a unique or controversial theoretical or clinical position.

We must now add to this discussion of the supervisor's roles in the training programs the role variations associated with beginning or more advanced clinicians. Not only is the supervisor expected to supervise every type of disorder, she is also expected to supervise students who are just beginning with the clinical experience, as well as students who are graduating with their master's degrees and ready to go into a CFY experience. The beginning clinician comes to the supervisor barely able to even recognize some types of disorders, having no background except lectures and, perhaps, never even having observed some types of disorders. To say the least, the supervisor's work is cut out for her. In this instance she must lead the clinician by the hand through the initial clinical experiences with the client. If the therapy is good, it is only because she told the clinician what to do and the clinician did exactly what she was told. The supervisor's job then is to get the beginning clinician to understand why she did what she did. The supervisor's role here is that of a lecturer, because she is involved in some very direct teaching.

At the other end of the continuum the supervisor is faced with the clinician who is at the end of her formal training. She has had many clinical experiences and been supervised by several supervisors. She has developed a good repertoire of skills and techniques and is gaining much insight into her therapy. The job of the supervisor now is to complete the clinical training by making certain that the clinician can supervise herself (self-supervision). The supervisor's role shifts here to that of a synthesizer, helping the clinician put her academic information and clinical knowledge together to focus on a problem. The supervisor is also a resource person, directing the clinician to sources of additional information that will assist in problem solving. She is a catalyst. She brings the clinician's problem-solving ability to the fore and shows the clinician not only how to resolve clinical problems but also what process she used to solve the problem. Once the clinician learns the process of solving clinical problems, she is ready for her professional exposure to therapy.

At an Internship Site

The supervisor's role in the agency that serves as an internship site is a bit less complex than that in the training program. The main reason for this is that she is supervising only more advanced clinicians. Although the criteria for being assigned to an internship may differ between training programs, a basic requirement of all programs is that the clinician demonstrate some clinical proficiency before being allowed to represent the training program at a professional agency. Because the reputation of the training program is at stake, the clinicians assigned to internships are carefully screened to make certain they will be good representatives for the program.

The clinician who has sufficient background to be assigned to an internship should not need the lecture approach by the supervisor except in those instances where she is confronted by disorder types she has never had experience with. Even in this instance, however, the clinician has a rather broad background of academic information and clinical experience to draw upon, so the supervisory informational meetings should go quite smoothly and rapidly. The supervisor is working with an advanced clinician and the main purpose of her supervision is to enhance and extend the self-supervision process that the clinician was taught by her supervisors in the training program.

There is again the question of what the supervisor should teach in terms of diagnostic and therapeutic approaches to disorder types. In that the supervisor is working within an independent agency, however, her problems with this issue are a bit different from the supervisor in the training program. If her agency advocates a particular approach to diagnostics and therapy for a disorder type, the decision is already made for the supervisor. She will teach the agency's approach. If the agency does not advocate any particular approach to a disorder type, the supervisor is free to teach her own approach. Because the clinician she is supervising is advanced, there will be less confusion as the supervisor departs from the faculty member's approach to the disorder and introduces her own. This will now add to the clinician's information about the disorder types, rather than create major confusion as it would for a beginning clinician.

At a Clinical Fellowship Year Site

The role of the supervisor is much more predictable in this environment. The clinician has now graduated from a training program and is embarking on her professional career. She comes into the site rather well prepared, having been supervised in both her training program and at one or more internships sites. She is prepared to work rather independently with a variety of cases. One might look at this supervision role as one of fine tuning the clinician. Supervision is less intense and the relationship between the supervisor and the clinician is one of professional colleagues sharing and discussing a client. The role of the supervisor is primarily that of a resource person, providing the clinician with highly specialized and unique informational resources.

In a Professional Setting

When a clinician begins working in a clinical environment that is unique to her, either in terms of the clinical approach used by the agency or in terms of the type of case load, she may be required to do some in-service training. This training will

NOTES

be supervised by another clinician in the agency. If the training is to introduce the clinician to a unique clinical approach, the supervisor will initially use the lecture technique as she introduces the new approach, and then will gradually shift her role to synthesizer and resource person. Her role as synthesizer is critical, because the clinician is experienced and has a great deal of information and clinical experience that needs to be focused on the new clinical approach to which she is being introduced. The supervisor's resource role is to provide published resources or materials. This information can then be synthesized by the clinician into the new clinical approach.

In the event that the clinical training is concerned with a unique clinical population, the same supervisory roles apply. The initial role is one of lecturer, as the supervisor introduces the clinician to the unique aspects of the clinical population. She also serves as a resource for the clinician. She provides, both in discussions and through resource materials, information that helps the clinician understand the uniqueness of the clinical population.

VARIATIONS IN THE ROLE OF THE SUPERVISEE

As a Trainee

The role of the student clinician in a training program is as varied as that of the supervisor. When the student first starts her clinical experience, her role with her supervisor is primarily as a student. She listens, thinks about what the supervisor says, and attempts to synthesize the information. If she comes to some conclusion about what has been said in the supervisory session, she shares this with her supervisor, not as a colleague but as a student sharing her opinion or thought. At this early point in clinical experience, the student clinician should have more questions than statements of opinion or thoughts. By the end of the clinical experience in the training program the role of the clinician changes rather dramatically. She should now be relating to the supervisor on a different level, one of sharing thoughts, ideas, and solutions to clinical problems she might be experiencing. The role shifts from that of a student to that of a new professional and her interaction with her supervisor changes from that of a student–teacher interaction to more of a peer relationship. She will have learned some self-supervision skills by this time, and her self-supervision now becomes the focus in her clinical conferences with her supervisor.

As a Clinical Fellowship Year Trainee

After graduation from a training program, the clinician enters a clinical fellowship year (CFY) in an agency where she performs as a professional clinician, but under the guidance of an experienced clinician, her clinical supervisor. Her role shifts again toward a more professional relationship with her supervisor. Conferences are now focused on the supervisor responding to questions and discussing the questions with the supervisee. In general, the clinical discussions are broad in nature, covering a wide range of clinical topics and issues.

As a Professional in a Unique Clinical Setting

Even though an individual may be a fully trained and qualified speech clinician or audiologist, there are still situations where she will need to receive "on-the-job training." This could involve a position as a clinician in an agency where the agency advocates a very specific form of treatment. The clinician must then be trained in the procedure and supervised as she learns to apply the procedure to clients. The role of the clinician is as a student, but her interaction with the supervisor is more of a peer relationship. Clinical conferences would consist of discussions between professionals, but the student–teacher relationship would also be present. These same roles would apply in the situation where the clinician joined an agency that dealt with a unique clinical population. If the clinician was not experienced with this population, she would receive specific training by a supervising clinician.

As the clinician in these situations becomes more familiar with either the clinical procedure or the population, her role shifts to that of a peer in her interactions with her supervisor. It would be assumed that the clinician had already developed her self-supervisory skills and that the in-service training would be short in duration.

As a Self-Supervisor

After learning the skills of self-supervision, the clinician has a very specific role to play in terms of evaluating her own clinical performance. This is the role of objective observer of her own therapy. She must be able to evaluate her own clinical behaviors in terms of their performance. She must also review her clinical progress with her clients and evaluate both the effectiveness and the efficiency of her treatment program. And, if there is a problem, she must be able to determine if it is a problem of the effectiveness of the program (where the client is not learning) or of the efficiency of the program (where learning is occurring but extremely slowly). She must first be able to determine where the problem is in the clinical process. She must see if the problem is with her overall plan, her interactions with the client, her clinical stimulus, her responses to the client, her behavioral-change goals, her client's attentiveness, or some other aspect of the clinical process. This is where the CIM provides the guidelines for problem solving. After determining what and where the problem is, she must be able to resolve the problem by making the necessary adjustments in her therapy. Her ability to perform self-supervision is directly related to her ability to remain objective as she evaluates her own clinical performance. The individual is truly a professional clinician only when she is able to self-supervise. A bit of a split personality comes in handy when attempting to create and maintain these two separate clinical roles.

NOTES

Cognitive Behavior Supervision

Chapter 4

The CBS Supervision Model: The SCIM

The CBS system is presented from the standpoint of its theoretical foundations, beginning with the Supervisory Transaction. The CIM is then reviewed and its role in the supervision conference (clinical teaching) is discussed. The CIM is then modified to the SCIM (Supervisory Clinical Interaction Model), which forms the basis of clinical teaching in the supervisory conference. The chapter is concluded with a discussion of the influence interpersonal relationships has on the supervisory process.

SUPERVISORY TRANSACTIONS

In Chapter 2 we established the clinician–client interactions as a series of transactions based on a stimulus-organism-response (S-O-R) exchange. The concept of the clinical transaction was developed into a model which was presented in Figure 2-1. Because interactions between the supervisor and the supervisee are also based on this S-O-R exchange, only minor modifications are necessary to make the original transaction model applicable to supervision. It is only necessary to change the two participants in the transactions, replacing "clinician" with "supervisor" and "client" with "supervisee." Thus, the first half of the transaction, S-O-R, represents the supervisor presenting the stimulus (S) to the supervisee, the organism (O), for cognition. The supervisee then provides the response (R) and the first half of the transaction is complete.

The second half of the transaction, S-O-R/<u>S-O-R</u>, represents the response of the supervisee becoming the stimulus (S) for the supervisor who, as the organism (O), evaluates the response and then responds (R) to the supervisee. This interaction constitutes one transaction. The next transaction builds on the results of this transaction. Each transaction is again dependent upon the previous transaction.

In the clinical conference each transaction constitutes a transfer of information, with the supervisor giving information to the supervisee or requesting information from her. The supervisor must determine basically if the information she sent was received properly and if the information she requested is correct. So, each transaction is tested by the supervisor after the supervisee has responded.

The supervisee's response, even when it is a question, provides the supervisor with insight into the status of the information that is being exchanged in the clinical conference. The supervisor needs to determine from the supervisee's response the correctness of the response, the depth and thoroughness of the response, the problem-solving process the supervisee used, and what the stimulus should be to start the next transaction. If the transaction has been successful, the supervisor rewards the supervisee and then moves ahead in the transactional process. However, if the transaction has not been successful, and the supervisee did not learn properly, the supervisor responds with a slight penalty, such as saying, "That's not quite right. Let me explain that again." She then repeats the transaction making a correction in her stimulus so it is more appropriate for the academic and clinical level of the supervisee.

THE ROLE OF THE SCIM IN THE SUPERVISION CONFERENCE

In Chapter 2, the CIM illustrated in detail the interactions between the clinician and the client. We now modify the model to the Supervisory Clinical Interaction Model (SCIM) so it applies to the interactions between the supervisee and the supervisor (See Figure 4-1). We will discuss the changes according to the supervisor's stimulus, cognitions, and response during the interaction.

The Supervisor's Stimulus (S)

The supervisor's stimulus, like the clinician's, is made up of modeling, guidance, and information. Although modeling was the most frequently used strategy by the clinician, it is not that useful to the supervisor. This does not mean that it is not used, but that its uses are limited. The supervisor may want to demonstrate the proper use of a diagnostic test, or demonstrate how the clinician should perform a model she is using in therapy. In order to do this, the supervisor will model the use of the test or the presentation of the stimulus. And, in an extreme case, she may even enter the therapy room as the clinician is engaged in therapy in order to model a teaching technique. However, there are a limited number of ways the supervisor can use modeling as a teaching strategy.

Guidance is also more limited in its use by the supervisor. She may use gestural guidance as she encourages the supervisee to continue with her analysis of a clinical situation, or she may combine gestural and verbal guidance to encourage the analysis. Verbal guidance might also be used in order to give more direct prompts to the supervisee as she attempts to resolve a clinical problem. For example, the supervisor might say, "You have now identified the two factors interfering with your therapy. I think I see some sort of relationship between the factors. Look at how they affect your client

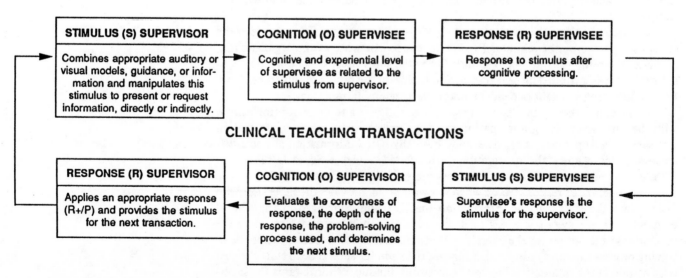

Figure 4-1. Supervisory Clinical Interaction Model (SCIM). This model, a modification of the original CIM model, illustrates the interactions taking place between the supervisor and the supervisee during clinical teaching. These interactions differ from clinical interactions in that they are almost exclusively focused on cognitive functions rather than on motor functions.

and tell me how you are going to deal with them." She would then gesture in such a way to cue the clinician to continue with her analysis.

The most important of the teaching strategies for the supervisor is giving information to and requesting it from the clinician. She provides the supervisee with information about such things as her clinical plan, her clinical performance, the type of client she is working with, her problem-solving strategies, and so forth. She also requests information to assess the supervisee's retention of information, the process of information recall, and the process used for problem solving. The focal point of the clinical conference is the exchange of information and the assessment of the supervisee's cognitions.

The Supervisee's Cognitions and Response (O-R/S)

The cognitive activity the supervisee engages in during any given transaction is dependent upon the supervisor's stimulus. If the supervisor is giving the supervisee information, the supervisee is thinking about information being presented, attempting to commit it to memory and trying to associate it with some relevant clinical factor such as the client she is working with, the type of test she is performing, and so forth. The cognitive function here is one of committing as much information as possible to memory.

This is also a "sorting and stacking" activity in which information is put into categories for storage and easy retrieval. No response is required here as long as the supervisor continues to give information or until she requests one. If the supervisor shifts her approach to the supervisee and instead of providing information requests information, the cognitive activity of the supervisee must shift from information storage to retrieval of stored information. In order to respond to the questions asked by the supervisor the supervisee must draw upon both her long- and short-term memory. The ability to retrieve stored information easily is critical, because clinical problem solving (self-supervision) is based on this. When a problem occurs during a transaction with a client, the clinician does not have unlimited time to ruminate about how to respond to the problem. This is why the sorting and stacking activity while storing information is so important. Any flaws in the storage system during this sorting and stacking cognitive activity create additional problems of comprehension or organization for the supervisee. This "disorganization" means that the supervisee cannot synthesize the available information into workable units, because some of the information does not seem appropriate. It is all traceable back to faulty sorting and stacking during the information storage. The resultant cognitive unrest prompts the supervisee to formulate questions to ask the supervisor to seek clarification of misunderstood information, or perhaps to distract the supervisor from the fact that she is completely confused. This could be the beginning of another game called "Let's Play 20 Questions."

Depending on the cognitive activity taking place in the conference, the supervisee has three basic responses to the supervisor. If the supervisor is providing information and then asking specific questions about what was said, such as, "What muscles are involved in this action?" the supervisee is expected to respond to the question. This verification-of-information exchange will give the supervisor some insight into how well the supervisee is receiving the information. The second response type is for the supervisee to answer a question that the supervisor directs to her but that is not directly related to information that has just been presented. This might be in response to the supervisor saying, "What do you think about that?"

The third response form, which might appear to be spontaneous but is really prompted directly or indirectly by the supervisor, is that of the supervisee asking questions of the supervisor. Although this situation might be interpreted as a reversal of

NOTES

roles in the transaction model, it actually continues to follow the model exactly. The supervisor sets the stage for a question period through her stimulus. For example she might say, "Do you have any questions about what I just said?" or a more generic, "Can I answer any questions you might have?" This may open a floodgate so most supervisors are leery of this open-ended statement. Some supervisees use this strategy to avoid discussions of their clinical prowess. This was discussed in Chapter 3.

The supervisee's response, whatever it is, becomes the stimulus for the supervisor. This is what she responds to. It is the supervisee's response that the supervisor analyzes to determine the focus of the next clinical transaction.

The Supervisor's Cognitions (O)

The first cognition the supervisor must perform is to estimate the cognitive knowledge level of the supervisee. This cognitive level is related to the supervisee's academic and clinical knowledge, and it establishes the level of the stimulus the supervisor will provide. This estimate may indeed be incorrect, either too high or too low, but the supervisor must establish a starting point. She may revise the estimate as she explores the supervisee's cognitions in each clinical transaction.

Each transaction must be tested before the next transaction can commence. The supervisor must determine if the transaction was successfully completed before she can move ahead in whatever activity she is engaged in. The type of testing the supervisor does depends on the purpose of the transaction. If the transaction is for providing the supervisee with some information, the supervisor must determine if the information was received correctly before proceeding to the next bit of information. After she has completed presenting an informational unit, she would then add a question to elicit a response from the supervisee. For example, the supervisor might say, "When you are attempting to teach your voice client an easy vocal attack, you must remember that there are two vocal fold positions involved in the problem. When the client produces a hard vocal attack, he first closes the vocal folds completely, and then tries to phonate. However, proper phonation is accomplished through approximation of the folds rather than vocal fold closure. Do you understand the difference between vocal fold closure and vocal fold approximation?" Thus, after she has given the supervisee the information on vocal attack, she then invites the supervisee to respond. When the supervisee responds, the supervisor can determine if she needs to repeat and expand on the information or if she can proceed to the next informational point she wants to make. It is only after the transaction has been completed and its success or failure determined that the supervisor can establish the direction of the next transaction. If the supervisee responds, "I thought the vocal folds had to be closed in order to produce phonation," the supervisor knows that the supervisee has a problem with the information she is trying to impart. In order to get this information across to the supervisee the transaction must be repeated and the stimulus modified to fit the cognitive knowledge level of the supervisee. Once the supervisee understands this information the supervisor can proceed with her presentation.

In another mode of testing, the supervisor asks the supervisee to resolve a hypothetical clinical problem. She gives the supervisee the necessary information about the situation and then asks, "As you know the client has a severe hearing loss and, due to cerebral palsy, also has problems with fine motor movements. How would you approach teaching this client to produce the [s] sound?" The supervisee is now called upon to utilize her academic and clinical knowledge (and her sorting and stacking) to solve the clinical problem. Her response will be the result of her cognitive evaluation of the problem and its apparent solution. The supervisor now evaluates the correctness of the response. She is not looking for a stock answer or the recitation of an answer from a reference book, but rather a response based on the cognitions of the supervisee, a response that indicates that she is thinking through the problem, calling on her knowledge and experience, and planning an appropriate approach to the problem. This is problem solving, the basis of self-supervision. The supervisor is looking both at the problem-solving process the supervisee used to reach her conclusions and the proposed resolution of the problem.

The final cognitive mode has to do with responding to questions asked by the supervisee. After inviting and receiving questions the supervisor must think not only of appropriate answers, but also must evaluate the quality of the questions themselves. She must determine if the questions reflect a severe lack of knowledge or confusion in the area or if this is just a minor point that can be cleared up by answering the question. She also needs to be aware of why the questions are being asked. Is this a true search for answers to questions or a ploy to gain attention, distract from other issues, or to try to impress her. When is a game a game?

After the supervisor makes a determination of the success or failure of the transaction, she then decides where the next transaction should go and how she should respond to the supervisee's response. If the supervisee clearly understands the information she has been presented, the supervisor rewards her by saying, "That's right. Very good." She then begins the next transaction with a stimulus that extends the information into the next phase. Each transaction repeats this process and is dependent upon the previous transaction to determine where it is going.

In a transaction where the purpose is problem solving, the supervisor evaluates the response of the supervisee both for the problem-solving process and the suggested resolution of the problem. However, if the problem-solving process is faulty, correct resolution of the clinical problem is almost impossible. So, if the suggested solution to the problem reflects faulty reasoning, the next transaction would focus on the problem-solving process. If both the process and the solution are acceptable, after some rewarding praise the next transaction would delve deeper into the problem.

The last situation concerns the supervisee asking questions of the supervisor. If the supervisor does not question the supervisee's motive or the reflected depth of knowledge, the supervisor might respond by saying, "The best way I can answer your question is...." However, if there is some evidence that there is a serious lack of knowledge in the subject matter, the supervisor might respond, "The question is a good one, but let me see if I can give you more general help in this area. Do you understand this concept...?" By asking a series of questions the supervisor can assess the supervisee's knowledge in the area and refocus the transactions on providing information that more directly addresses an informational deficit, rather than responding to a series of questions. The questions will, more than likely, not focus on the deficit, as it appears the supervisee does not even know that she does not know.

The Supervisor's Response (R)

It is extremely important for the supervisor to respond to the supervisee at the end of each transaction. There is no better way to discourage motivation and interest than to ignore the responses of the supervisee. There are only two ways the supervisor can respond; with either a positive response (which takes on the characteristics of a reward) or a negative response (a penalty). We are taking the position here that there is no such thing as a totally neutral response. Each response takes on, to some degree, either positive or negative characteristics. Constructive criticism, often sold to unsuspecting recipients as a form of reward, is actually a form of penalty that is prettied up so it looks like something positive. It contains a double message, as does being reprimanded by someone who has a smile on her face. It fools no one, particularly when it is given by a supervisor. It is a form of judgment, and the judgment is that the performance was not adequate. As long as we recognize constructive criticism for what it really is, we can deal with it.

One of the most common forms of reward from a supervisor is the phrase, "That's good," or just, "Good." After the supervisee has heard it several times, it becomes meaningless. How many times can someone say, "Good," to you before it becomes just a word? All supervisees who are reading this should stop and think of how this works as a reward in therapy; about as well as it works with you in your conference with your supervisor. Come to think of it, this may be where all supervisors learn to reward by saying, "Good," or, "That's good."

Rewards for the supervisee should be of a social nature, actions or words on the part of the supervisor that are social in nature and convey approval. The challenge for the supervisor is to come up with forms of approval that are clear to the supervisee and do not fade to the point where they are meaningless.

Even though most supervisors may deny using penalty as a teaching tool, it is an integral part of almost every supervisory conference. Penalty may take the form of a frown on the supervisor's face as the supervisee is presenting her solution to a clinical problem. Or it may be the supervisor saying, "Well, that's not quite right." Some people call this negative feedback, but it is just penalty packaged under a different label. Penalty is anything that the supervisee finds even slightly aversive, and it is a very powerful teaching tool. When used in conjunction with reward the combination is almost unbeatable.

THE SUPERVISEE'S RESPONSE TO REWARDS AND PENALTIES

Everyone likes to be rewarded, even supervisees. And when the supervisee likes the reward and wants more of it, she develops approach motivation. She is motivated to perform those behaviors that result in rewards, because she wants the rewards. Motivation is an extremely important attitude in supervisees, because it leads to creative activity. Approach motivation is one of the most powerful factors operating in good clinicians. They want to receive rewards not only from the supervisor, but also from the sense of accomplishment in their clinical interactions with their clients. One of the most efficient ways to destroy motivation is to ignore the supervisee's efforts to function adequately in the clinical environment.

Supervisees also have a reaction to penalty. They, like all people, want to avoid penalty. When they discover what it is that they do to provoke the penalty, they will attempt to avoid doing that thing. Extremely subtle use of penalty can be devastating to supervisees because, in many instances, they cannot identify what behavior is being penalized. When the supervisee knows exactly what she is penalized for, she develops avoidance motivation, motivation not to perform the penalized activity so she can avoid the penalty.

When approach motivation is combined with avoidance motivation, learning becomes very efficient and effective. Consider the following situation. The supervisee is performing behavior X and the supervisor finds the behavior a serious impediment to therapy. So, the supervisor guides the supervisee to perform behavior Y which, when substituted for behavior X, makes therapy more efficient. Now, in order to get the new behavior occurring quickly in therapy she rewards the supervisee for performing behavior Y (increasing the frequency of its occurrence) and at the same time penalizes occurrences of X (decreasing the frequency of its occurrence). Thus, not only is the supervisor using the supervisee's approach motivation to encourage the performance of behavior Y, she is also using her avoidance motivation to discourage the performance of behavior X. This is an example of the carrot and the stick philosophy; dangle a carrot in front of the mule to entice him to move ahead, but have a big stick behind him to encourage movement from that end. If it works with mules and with clients, why not with supervisees?

THE INFLUENCE OF INTERPERSONAL RELATIONSHIPS IN SUPERVISION

There are two very important words, or concepts, to consider here. Although they may appear to represent the same concept, they are as different as apples and applesauce. The words are *like* and *respect*.

When we say we "like" someone, we are saying that we enjoy the person, we enjoy being with the person. When we are with the person we are relaxed and at ease, because the person does not threaten us. There are many people we like and we consider these people our "friends."

When we consider the word "respect" we are talking about admiration and esteem. We look with wonder on the person we admire and respect. We might even be a bit intimidated by the person, because we admire his or her accomplishment or station in life. We often respect a position, such as a public official, even though we do not actually respect or admire the person holding the office.

If we think of our friends we will find that, with some, we both like and respect them. You not only enjoy being around them, but you also admire and respect them. However, there are also those friends we like but do not particularly respect: "Bob is really a joy to be around but he is totally unreliable. You can never count on him for anything." Then there are the people we respect but do not like. We do not consider these people our friends because liking a person is essential to friendship. Perhaps they are egotistical, or hard to get along with, or remote, but they have earned our respect in one way or another. Perhaps you can think of one of your former professors who fits this description.

So, there are three basic types of relationships: one in which you like the other person, one in which you respect the other person, and one where you both like and respect the other person. In our society today, and even in our profession, being liked by others has taken on disproportionate significance. Many people will not take an unpopular stance on an issue because, if they do it, others will not like them. And many clinicians make this their first and only priority in their relations with their clients. We would suggest that the most important ingredient in a clinical relationship is being respected, not liked. Of course the combination of being liked and respected by the client makes the best possible clinical relationship, but if this is not attainable, the clinician should work toward being respected by the client.

These same general rules of interpersonal relationships apply to the relationships between supervisors and supervisees. And the rules apply both ways in this relationship. The supervisor must like, respect, or like and respect the supervisee. If none of this is present in the relationship, if the supervisor dislikes and has no respect for the supervisee, there can be little profitable interaction, and the supervisee will learn nothing from the supervisor. All supervisors have worked with supervisees whom they did not particularly like, but they had to respect that fact that they were students studying under them, and as such they should be shown common courtesy and respect. There is never any cause for a supervisor to be disrespectful to a supervisee.

The supervisee will also form an opinion of the supervisor. She may like the supervisor but have no respect for her or her advice. Or she may not particularly like the supervisor but have great respect for her clinical teaching. The best combination for both parties is for the supervisee to both like and respect the supervisor. If this feeling is mutual, it will lead to good clinical teaching.

These interpersonal relationships have a profound effect on the motivation of the supervisee. If the supervisee does not like or respect the supervisor, she will not be motivated to do her best work for her. She may perform to get a grade, but this is not a good mental set for learning. And, if there is actual animosity between the supervisor and supervisee, it will have a negative effect on the learning, with the supervisee rejecting the advice and suggestions of the supervisor.

Each of these parties, the supervisor and the supervisee, has an obligation to develop the best possible relationship for the teacher–learner interaction. Perhaps honesty is the one ingredient that will make this relationship viable. Hidden agendas, manipulations, game playing, and other such items do not lead to good interpersonal relationships, which are the very soul of the clinical conferences. A good learning experience can only occur in an environment that is learning oriented, not confrontational.

Chapter 5

Data Collection for Supervision

In order for the supervisor to evaluate the supervisee's performance, she must collect data on that performance. The methods available to the supervisor are written information, clinical observations, and the supervisory conference itself. The purpose of data collection, to assess the academic and clinical levels of the clinician to determine where improvement is needed, is discussed in terms of its forming the base of the clinical teaching in the supervisory process.

INTRODUCTION

Although this chapter might appear to be directed only to the clinical supervisor, it is also directed to the supervisee; she too is responsible for supervising her clinical performances. She must also collect data on her performance in order to evaluate it. She has two supervisors or clinical teachers; her regular clinical supervisor and herself.

Clinical teaching is dependent on detailed data collection. The supervisor must have exact data collected on the performance of the supervisee before there can be a teaching–learning interaction. She must establish the behavioral proficiency level of the supervisee in order to assess performance, and take steps then to improve the supervisee's clinical performance. Data are collected from three main sources: written materials, clinical observations, and clinical conferencing.

WRITTEN INFORMATION

Each training program or agency has its own required written materials. We will discuss the three general areas we feel are common to most programs or agencies.

Reports

Reports can be made on a variety of subjects, but we are focusing on the diagnostic report, clinical progress reports, and the end-of-the-term report. As the supervisor reviews these reports she can assess not only the supervisee's writing style and ability, she can also gather data on the amount and type of information the supervisee has available, and how well she is able to synthesize this information into a report that is professional, understandable, and logical in its presentation of materials.

The amount of information available to the supervisee is somewhat dependent on her academic and clinical levels. Not only does the clinician gain additional academic information as she progresses through her training program, she also gains, from her clinical experience, the ability to utilize this information in her therapy and her written reports. More writing experience, coupled with editing by the supervisor and rewriting exercises, improves her writing proficiency so that she includes more information in her reports and that information is better synthesized and reported in a clearer style. The supervisee's progress in gaining information and utilizing it in problem solving is manifested in all of her report writing. This is a major source of data for the supervisor.

We will only mention the supervisees' spelling in passing. It is a universal problem, partially because English has borrowed so many foreign words, retaining the original spelling but changing the pronunciation. English is not a phonetically based language. This may explain why so many students have trouble getting through their phonetics course. This may also explain why there are so many dictionaries. The problem with the dictionary, however, is that if you do not know how to spell the word it is almost impossible to look it up to find how to spell it.

Lesson Plans

There is no better way for the supervisor to gather data about the supervisee's clarity of thought and utilization of information than from the lesson plan. Lesson plans offer the supervisor a different type of data—data directly related to the immediate clinical situation the supervisee faces. The supervisee is able to write a good lesson plan only if she can use the information she has been given on the disorder type. The supervisee must also understand the logical sequence of therapy for the particular disorder. If she does not have this information, there will be no logical sequencing either within each lesson plan or between lesson plans.

Self-Evaluations

Self-evaluations can also be a valuable source of information about the supervisee. However, the self-evaluation can be misleading if the supervisee is either not aware of her clinical strengths and weaknesses or is attempting to manipulate the supervisor with a game.

If the supervisee is truly unaware of her strengths and weaknesses, this factor in itself is of extreme importance to the supervisor. The factor increases in importance in direct relationship to the level of experience of the supervisee. The supervisor might not expect a beginning level clinician to have insights into her inadequacies, but if this situation continues in an intermediate level clinician, a serious problem is emerging. If the supervisee does not have this insight into her own performance she will not be able to do any meaningful problem solving. Because problem solving is the basis of self-supervision, she will not be able to perform this necessary clinical function. The clinician cannot progress to the advanced and professional levels until this problem has been rectified. This lack of awareness is directly related to the supervisee's sensitivity to the existence of problems in her therapy. Thus, the clinician's self-evaluations are an extremely valuable source of information for the supervisor.

OBSERVATIONS

Observation of the supervisee in the clinical environment is the best source of data for the supervisor. This type of data is directly related to the supervisee's performance of clinical behaviors. The clinical interaction with the client represents the synthesis of all the clinician's academic knowledge, clinical experience, and all of the previous supervisory discussions and conferences into a single performance. It is the performance that demonstrates how well the supervisee is able to incorporate her knowledge, experience, and cognitions into interactions with a client. It is the proficiency of the performance that forms the basis of the next conference between the supervisor and the supervisee.

Observations of clinical interactions can be either direct observations through one-way mirrors or while sitting in the therapy room with the supervisee, or indirect observations by viewing a scene of ongoing therapy or a videotaped recording of previous therapy. Observation through a one-way mirror yields the best observational data. Sitting in the therapy room with the clinician and the client creates too many problems. It is not a viable option, unless there are extenuating circumstances, such as there being no other means of observation.

The video picture of ongoing therapy has only one advantage, that being that the supervisor does not have to go and sit behind a one-way mirror. But this mode of observation has many disadvantages, such as a restricted view of therapy and loss of detail in what is seen. The recorded videotape of therapy has the same disadvantages but it does have two redeeming features. First of all, the clinician is able to observe herself in the clinical interaction. This is invaluable, because the supervisee can more or less objectively witness her performance. And then there is instant replay; the supervisor can make the supervisee watch her mistake over and over again until she understands what she did that was wrong. The supervisee can also watch her finest hour over and over, if indeed there was such a session and if it was recorded (but, we all know that only the "bad" sessions are recorded for analysis by the supervisor).

We feel that the best possible observations are those that take place live with the supervisor seated behind the one-way mirror taking in the whole clinical scene. The second best mode of observation is watching a video recording of therapy, the unique strength here being the ability to demonstrate behaviors for the supervisee. The least desirable is observing ongoing therapy through a television monitor. This last mode does not show enough clinical detail, especially if the supervisor is going to base a grade on the observation.

There are two general purposes of an observation: observation for general data gathering, and observation for data gathering upon which to base an evaluation. General observations might be considered an overview of the clinician–client interaction, a molar view as opposed to a molecular view. The supervisor might not even take a note during the observation, depending rather on her ability to form a general impression of the clinical proficiency of the supervisee. This type of observation can be made by observing therapy on a video monitor since fine details are not needed. These clinical impressions, however, influence future observations where the supervisee is being evaluated.

In the evaluative observation the supervisor is observing specific behavioral performances and rating each performance on some evaluative scale. Performances are rated against a clinical behavioral standard and the ratings are then translated into a grade for clinical performance. This type of observation should be done directly by watching the clinical interaction from behind a one-way mirror. In most video systems the camera is positioned for the best view of the entire clinical scene, which does not allow the supervisor to observe subtle details in interactions.

We must also consider the auditory "observation," the listening to an audiotape of the therapy interaction. This is the least desirable and least productive form of observation, but it is also the most common form available to the supervisee as she evaluates her own therapy. In this mode, much of the context of the verbal interaction is lost. The listener can hear all of the content of the interchange, but can only assume the context of the interchange. The data collected from this observation are very limited, and the reliability and validity of the data without visual validation are always in question. This mode should be used by the supervisor only when no other form of observation is available. When the supervisee uses audio recordings of her clinical session

NOTES

for observation, she should remember the problems of reliability and validity of the data collected. We do not mean to infer that this is not a valuable source of data for the supervisee, only that she should be aware of the limitations of the data.

THE SUPERVISION CONFERENCE

After the supervisor has collected her data she has a conference with the supervisee. The conference interaction is illustrated in the SCIM (see Figure 4-1). This interaction provides the supervisor with a splendid opportunity to gather more data. However, these data are not related to the clinical behaviors, but rather to the status of the supervisee's store of academic information, the amount of clinical experiential information, insights she has into the interactions between these information banks, and the problem-solving cognitive processes she uses in bringing these sources of information together in the conference. If the clinical observational data form the basis of evaluation of behavioral performance, the conference data form the basis of evaluation of cognitive performance. The cognitive data are used to shape the supervisee's cognitive processes so that she is able to recognize and solve clinical problems that will confront her in professional life. Without the problem-solving cognitive skill there can be no self-supervision. And without self-supervision, there is no professional growth.

During the conference the supervisor must make note not only of the effectiveness of the supervisee's cognitive processing, but also the depth, or lack of depth, of academic information. Both of these factors are reflected in the answers the supervisee gives and in the questions that she asks in the conference. The data the supervisor gathers in this contact can be used to direct the supervisee to outside readings to make up for some academic deficits, to direct the supervisee to have a conference with the teaching faculty member whose area of expertise is in the area of the deficit, or to "lecture" the supervisee on the deficit area.

If the data collection indicates that the information is present but the cognitive sorting and stacking processing is weak or poorly organized, the supervisor can assist the supervisee by either leading her through a proper cognitive approach to an issue or to attempt to explain the process to her. One way the supervisor might approach this weakness in cognitive processing would be to have the supervisee hand in her written reports and lesson plans in outline form, thus forcing her to organize her thoughts in a logical sequence.

We are certain that there are other sources for data collection by the supervisor. We have only considered the most obvious ones that are common to programs where there is supervision. Regardless of where the data come from, the purpose remains the same; to improve the clinical and cognitive skills of the supervisee.

Chapter 6

Operational Definitions of Clinical Behaviors

A good treatment program is dependent upon the performance of a series of clinical behaviors. There are several categories of the 43 behaviors set forth in the CBS system as necessary for an effective and efficient treatment program. The categories are Planning, Interactions, Management, Procedures, Diagnosis, and Additional Clinical Responsibilities. Within each category, each behavior is operationally defined, with clinical examples in many of the definitions. All behavioral descriptions are numbered for convenient reference from all evaluation forms.

BEHAVIORAL ORIENTATION

What is ideal therapy? This is a question that the clinical supervisor must ask herself each time she supervises. The ideal is the standard that supervisors use for comparison when rating a clinician's performance. As they observe the clinical interactions between the clinician and the client, they must make a decision as to how the therapy they are supervising compares to this ideal therapy. Logically, this standard tends to be their own therapy, because this is the only therapy that they completely understand and most often approve of. Each clinician's therapy is a matter of pride, because it is a very personal endeavor. This is the ultimate expression of their knowledge, their personality, and their professionalism. If they do not have pride in their own therapy, they do not have pride in their profession. Therefore, each supervisor has her own concept of the best possible approach to a clinical situation; her own approach. Because each supervisor has a unique training and clinical background, is there any wonder then that there is a lack of consistency between supervisors?

The clinical interactions that are supervised are very complex. Some supervisors judge them on a "gestalt" basis, taking in the entire process and then reacting to it as an overall entity. Terms used to describe this approach include *molar*, to indicate the overview or "whole" approach. The opposite of this is *molecular*, which refers to attending to the parts that make up the whole. The problem with the molar view is that the supervisors using this approach have few, if any, specific suggestions on how to improve the therapy interaction, because they are attending only to the whole, not to the parts.

The other side of this coin, the molecular view, is more common among clinical supervisors. Here the concern is with the parts as they combine to constitute the whole. The major point of conjecture here is what constitutes the parts. Where there is no standard definition of the parts that make up the whole, each supervisor creates in her mind what parts are necessary and how the parts must be performed to create ideal therapy. There is little agreement among the various supervisors who create this ideal, because each comes from a different clinical background with different clinical experiences, which serve as reference points to create the parts which make up the

NOTES

ideal whole. In case you feel that there is much ambiguity here, you are correct. The parts are not well defined, they are not categorized, the criteria for excellence in performance are not set forth, and there is little agreement among supervisors. Thus, the supervisee receives mixed messages from her various supervisors, different parts being important to, and different criteria for excellence being set forth by each. Perhaps this makes it a bit easier to understand the game, "But Ms. Smith Liked it That Way." This is not always a game. In many, if not most instances, this is fact not fiction, and the clinician is simply pleading for some sort of agreement between supervisors.

In creating the CBS system we recognize that a standard for ideal therapy is crucial for the supervisor. To do this, the parts of this ideal therapy must be clearly set forth and defined so that each supervisor has the same basic information as she creates her ideal standard. That, then, is the purpose of this chapter, to set forth the molecular parts of the molar ideal clinical interaction.

In order to set forth these molecular parts as clearly as possible we turn to a behavioral approach that allows us to be very specific in terms of which behaviors constitute the molecular underpinnings of therapy. We view behavior as a physiological event, something that a clinician does. It is not necessarily a single event, such as clarifying goals for each clinical session (see Behavior 22, page 59) but could also consist of a series of individual behaviors which results in a more molar behavioral event, such as making therapy a time-efficient procedure (see Behavior 27, page 61). We even view cognition as a behavior, because it is a physiological event that, we hope, the clinician performs on a regular basis during therapy.

By using specific behaviors as the molecular units that make up the molar unit called therapy, we can operationally define them. The supervisor can then synthesize these behavioral entities into her molar view of ideal therapy that she uses as her standard in supervision.

This chapter is devoted to clarifying those behaviors considered crucial by the CBS system for satisfactory clinical performance. The creation of the instruments and list of clinical behaviors spanned the 50 combined years of our experience as supervisors, and were over two years in planning and development. The clinical behaviors associated with the system that are deemed essential for good therapy were selected with great care and only after consulting a wide variety of sources. In addition to our own choices of behaviors, we depended on recommendations from the clinical supervisors who were testing the system in the various training programs. We also discussed the choice of clinical behaviors with a number of highly experienced clinicians and clinical supervisors in a variety of professional settings. We reviewed the literature in supervision and more general professional books to find further suggestions of clinical behaviors. The position statement regarding supervision in *Asha* (1985) was also a source we investigated. Finally, many clinical behaviors were suggested in the chapter on cognitive behavior therapy, more specifically the CIM, in *The Handbook of Clinical Methods in Communication Disorders* (Leith, 1984).

The CBS system has identified and defined 43 behaviors that should occur when engaging in all aspects of clinical functioning. These behaviors, on which the supervisee will be rated, are divided into several distinct categories. The first category, Planning, includes those behaviors that occur prior to the session as the clinician prepares for therapy. These preparations include developing long- and short-range goals, as well as planning for implementation of session objectives. The second category, Interactions, includes those behaviors that are expected to occur in the supervisee's relationships with clients, parents, and supervisors. The third category, Management, includes behaviors that are related to maintaining client behavior and motivation. The fourth category, Procedures, includes those behaviors that occur during the session which are related to the therapeutic process.

Even though many behaviors included in each of these four categories apply to the diagnostic process, additional behaviors specific to diagnosis are identified and included under a separate heading, Diagnosis. Additionally, there are a number of other clinical behaviors that do not fall in any of the designated categories and are not assessed until the middle or end of the term. These behaviors are labeled Additional Clinical Responsibilities, and include such things as following clinic policies and the ability to self-supervise.

It is important for the supervisor and supervisee to have a mutual understanding of the specific behaviors that will be assessed. The remainder of this chapter will include discussion and definitions of each of the 43 clinical behaviors identified in the CBS supervision system.

NOTES

BEHAVIORAL DESCRIPTORS BY CATEGORIES

Planning

1. Formulates Long-Term Goals

Long-term goals are those goals the clinician expects the client to achieve within a specific time frame; for example, the goals expected to be reached during a semester in a clinical practicum. It is important to plan long-term goals when developing a treatment program for a client, because if the long-term goals are not established, the logical sequence of short-term goals cannot be formulated. It is important that the clinician, in formulating long-term goals, demonstrate insight and understanding of her client and the particular disorder being manifested. Goals should be comprehensive and appropriate for both the client and disorder. If goals appear to be in conflict with goals normally associated with a particular disorder, this conflict should be acknowledged and justified. Because long-term goals are the foundation of a treatment program, great care should be taken in explaining the rationale for the unique goal and how therapy planning is affected. The severity of the disorder manifested by the client should also be taken into consideration. Additionally, any associated behaviors the client might have, such as a lower cognitive functioning level, visual and auditory perceptual difficulties, or disturbances in motor functioning, should also be considered in planning. Long-term goals should be attainable within the time frame of the clinical experience. They should be written using behavioral terminology that describes the conditions under which the behavior should occur, how often it will be expected to occur, and how it will be evaluated in terms of frequency of occurrence and quality of performance.

2. Formulates Objectives Session by Session

The session objectives are a reflection of the clinical progress toward the long-term goals. The objectives should outline a logical sequence of clearly defined measurable behaviors which are valid in relation to the long-term goals. The clinician should state objectives in terms of client performance, using behavioral terminology and including methods to measure behavioral progress toward the objectives.

As with long-term goals, the objectives should be appropriate for the particular disorder, age, and interests of the client and relevant to the client's environment. Objectives should be attainable in the allotted time, but challenging enough to maintain client interest and motivation.

The session objectives should reflect adjustments that must be made in the treatment sequence due to client successes or failures during the previous session. By formulating objectives for each clinical session, the clinician is keeping close track of the client's clinical progress, which increases her sensitivity to clinical problems. It also assists her in solving clinical problems that arise, because she has a record over time of the progress the client has made.

The clinician should be sensitive to the need to modify objectives when either the objectives have been met or when it is deemed that sufficient time has been spent in unsuccessful attempts to achieve an objective. If the objective has been met, the clinician should create a new objective that is the next logical step in achieving the long-term goal. This change should be done as soon as the original objective is achieved so that the natural flow of clinical progress toward the long-term goal is not interrupted. The clinician should also be aware of client frustration if he is unable to achieve the planned objective. It is important that she recognize that continued failure on the part of the client is detrimental to his motivation and the resultant frustration is counterproductive to clinical progress. In this event she should make an adjustment in the clinical objective according to the skill level of the client.

A common planning error, especially with beginning-level clinicians, is in failing to differentiate between clinical procedures—objectives a clinician has planned for herself—and the behavioral objectives set forth for the client. In a supervision conference the supervisor and supervisee may have determined a need for the clinician to plan activities that would elicit more verbal responses from the client. A behavioral objective for the session, however, would not be to "participate in experiential play activities" or even "to increase verbal responses." Rather, the session objective should specify the type and frequency of the responses expected from the client.

3. Modifies the Clinical Program When Change is Indicated

The clinician's long-term and short-term planning typically center around a particular clinical method or program. There are times when that method or program should be modified, and the clinician needs to be able to recognize when change is indicated. When the client's performance levels have reached a plateau and no further progress is being made with the present program, this should be a signal to the clinician to make the appropriate changes. Another indicator that change is needed would be when a particular approach does not appear to be effective with a particular client. There are also times when changes in the client's physical, mental, or medical condition directly affect the disorder and necessitate program modification. When any change in the clinical program is indicated, the clinician should be able to make the modifications, including the development of new long- and short-term objectives when appropriate.

4. Materials Appropriate for Client

The choice of materials for therapy is an important consideration. The right materials can assist in creating interest in therapy and in achieving and maintaining approach motivation. However, if they are selected without considering the needs of the client and the type of disorder being worked with, the materials can work against the clinician by voiding any interest the client might have and, perhaps, even creating avoidance motivation. For this reason the clinician must demonstrate some clinical insight in the choice of materials for therapy. Materials should be stimulating enough to attract the client's attention and interesting enough to be motivating. Variables that the clinician should take into consideration when selecting materials are the age of the client, the sex of the client, the disorder the client manifests, the client's visual and auditory perceptual abilities, the cognitive level of the client, the client's motor skill level, and the client's interests. Only by considering these factors can the clinician fit the materials to the individual client. Keep in mind that the materials are chosen to maintain the interest and attention of the client, not the clinician.

The selection of the appropriate materials may have a bearing on how well the clinician can achieve Clinical Behavior 6 (Structures Plan for Maximum Number of Responses). If the selected material is a game with rather complicated directions, or the activity includes making something that requires considerable physical manipulation (such as cutting, gluing, or coloring), then client response time may be diminished, negatively effecting Clinical Behavior 32 (Client Talking/Response Time).

We view planning and preparing the materials as a separate skill from the actual use of them in the therapy session. It has been our experience that many clinicians are able to plan what should be very effective and motivating materials but, because of other technical difficulties, cannot efficiently implement the use of the material during the session.

Selection of materials for a conference is also important. Well designed charts to demonstrate progress, examples of the client's work, and copies of reports or tests which have been administered might all be helpful in a conference with a significant other (or even a clinical supervisor).

5. Has Rationale for Clinical Procedures

There is no single clinical procedure for any type of client. Essentially, the clinician is free to use any clinical procedure she feels is appropriate for the client and the disorder. However, the clinician also needs to have a rationale for her selection of the procedure. The rationale should be based on factual information gathered from research findings, clinical reports, classroom lecture notes, conferences, or from some other reliable source. The clinician should also understand why the selected procedure will likely succeed with this particular client and disorder. She should be able to communicate the rationale and reasons for its selection to the supervisor. Incorporated in her planning of therapeutic or diagnostic procedures should be a demonstrated understanding of the theoretical base of the CIM. If the clinician does not understand the theory underlying the CIM, she will not be able to plan appropriate procedures. If procedures are not appropriate, the therapeutic or diagnostic interaction with the client will fail.

6. Structures Plan for Maximum Number of Responses

In order for learning to occur in the clinical environment the client must be able to respond, to try to perform the behavior being taught or to respond verbally to see if a new concept or skill has been learned. The more chances the client has to perform and practice the new behavior, the quicker learning occurs. The clinician's therapy plan should reflect this concept, making certain that the client has enough opportunities to respond. Planned activities should require responses from the client, and there should be enough time allowed for the client to respond appropriately. Activities during which both the client and the clinician are silent, or where the client is only listening, should be held to a minimum. Rewards planned for therapy should not consume valuable clinical time in their administration or, in the case where edibles are used, in their consumption. The plan should reflect an attempt by the clinician to maximize the opportunities for the client to respond, as well as the responses by the client.

It should be obvious from the plan that the clinician has thought through carefully what she will do to help the client respond. Plans that include terms such as "establishing rapport," "discussion," and "talk about" are vague, which may allow the client and clinician to get off target.

7. Demonstration of Progress to the Client

In planning therapy, the clinician should always include some means of demonstrating progress to her client. In any learning situation, the learner must know where he is and where he needs to go in mastering the target behavior. He also needs to know of his progress as he moves closer and closer to achieving the goal. This awareness of progress is essential for interest and motivation, which are both essential for learning. This feedback keeps the learner on track, moving him step by step toward mastery of the goal behavior. The clinician should plan a means of demonstrating progress that is appropriate for the client. She should take into consideration how often the feedback should occur and what type should be used. The method should be clinically sound and easily provided so that it is effective and efficient. It should also provide for demonstration of improvement in behavioral performance over time.

8. Significant Others Included in Therapy Plan

This may not apply with some adult clients where there is little reason to include significant others or where there are no significant others to include. In the main, however, with either adults or children, the clinician should plan to include significant others in some aspect of the therapy, be it for moral support during therapy or for carryover of the new behavior into external environments. In the case of an adult client, the involvement of significant others in therapy is an individual and agency matter that must be determined and justified by the clinician. With children there are instances or settings, such as a public school, where the significant others (especially parents) are not readily available to participate actively in the therapy program. However, even in this situation, significant others must be appraised of the clinical findings in the diagnostic evaluation and of the therapy plan if treatment is indicated. There are some treatment plans that are dependent on cooperation from significant others and the clinician should address this dependency in her treatment plan and set forth alternatives if the cooperation of significant others diminishes.

The clinician should be aware that for some clients there may be persons other than a spouse or parent who may be in the role of significant other. These may be siblings, friends, a teacher, or a "speech buddy" in the therapy group. Through careful planning, significant others can be systematically included in either the therapy sessions or generalization activities.

Although in many situations there will be numerous opportunities for informal follow up or suggestions to significant others, it is important to provide more formal opportunities for gaining their support. Examples might include:

- Using a speech notebook or folder for the client to use between sessions to practice with a significant other
- Providing written suggestions of the "how to help" variety, or copies of useful articles or pamphlets regarding the client's problem
- Sending periodic progress notes or report cards to significant others
- Providing incentives for charting practice time between sessions

Interactions: Clinical and Supervisory

9. Sensitivity/Awareness

Throughout either the diagnostic or clinical session the clinician needs to have a heightened awareness of the client. She needs to be sensitive to both direct comments by the client and to subtle clues that indicate interest, motivation, feelings, needs, and so forth. This information may be goal-related, such as indicating that the client is meeting an objective or that more instruction is needed, or it may be related to how the client is feeling, physically or emotionally. This awareness on the part of the clinician should influence her therapeutic interactions and how she responds to meet her client's needs. Her awareness and perception of the client's signals are essential if she is to respond appropriately. She has to adjust her therapy to the attitudes and needs of the client if clinical progress is to be made.

10. Relates to the Client as a Person

In a humanistic approach to therapy the clinician treats her client as a human being and not, as in a technical or mechanical approach, as a subject in an experiment. The clinician should relate to her clients with dignity and respect, demonstrating unconditional positive regard. If the clinician interacts with an adult aphasic client as she would with a child, this will have an adverse effect on the client's attitude toward therapy. The clinician should also demonstrate to the client that she is sincerely interested in the client as an individual, not just interested in the communication disorder. Her focal point in the clinical interaction is on the client, not on the clinical procedure, method, or strategy.

If the clinician has no regard for a client as an individual, it will have a negative impact on her interactions with the client. It is important for the clinician to control her prejudices and biases. For example, she must relate with equal warmth and caring to a child who is dirty and poorly dressed as to the child from the affluent family who is always clean and wears designer clothes.

11. Affect in Therapy

The clinician should recognize that her attitude or cognitive set in a clinical interaction will have a direct influence on the attitude or cognitive set of the client or significant other. If she is enthusiastic about what she is doing, others coming in contact with her will more than likely also be enthused. She should appear to enjoy the experience, and chances are her client will too. She should demonstrate sincerity in her relations with her client or significant others by exhibiting a relaxed and caring attitude in the clinical setting. If the client perceives therapy in light of these positive clinician attitudes, he likely will be more positive himself and have more approach motivation in therapy. If the significant other perceives that the clinician is a sincere, caring individual, they too will be more responsive in the clinical interaction.

12. Negative Personal Factors Removed from Therapy

The secret to good interpersonal relations is to keep one's own negative feelings and personal problems from interfering with the relationship. We can only do this by making a concerted effort to block them from surfacing. The clinician should keep her personal attitudes, feelings, and beliefs out of her clinical interactions. The most important thing is that she recognize her own biases. If she does not recognize and then control her personal biases, they will show in her interactions with her clients. If her biases are negative, her relationships will deteriorate to the point where therapy is impossible. There are also personal factors that distract the clinician from therapy. In the case of student clinicians, there may be numerous distractions, such as worrying about an upcoming test to having done poorly in a class. With all clinicians there are personal problems, such as the ending of a romance, a fight with a boyfriend or husband, problems with children, a dent in the car, an overdrawn checking account, and so on. However, no matter what the problem is, the client's therapy should not suffer. In a case where a problem such as a death or serious illness of a family member might hamper the clinician's effectiveness, the clinician should take the appropriate steps to see that necessary arrangements are made. These should be consistent with the agency's policies and procedures.

13. Initiative/Independence

The end result of the supervision process should be clinician self-supervision. The foundation of self-supervision is initiative and independent problem solving by the clinician. When problems or questions arise, the clinician should demonstrate initiative and make an attempt to find answers before seeking help from the supervisor. She should have alternative solutions prepared when going in for a supervisory conference. As the clinician gains knowledge and experience she should become more independent in both recognizing problems and seeking solutions.

14. Confident Image in Clinical Setting

When a person is involved in working with others in any helping profession, the recipient of the aid must have confidence in the individual providing the aid. Confidence and credibility go hand in hand; and clinical credibility is an essential part of therapy. Hence, the clinician should make a positive professional impression on her clients and their significant others. She should instill confidence in them, confidence that she is a competent clinician and knowledgeable about the diagnosis and treatment of the client's particular communication disorder. Her confidence should be obvious in her posture, her facial expressions, her dress, and her speech. We do not mean to imply that a student clinician or even a practicing professional will, or should, know all the answers to all the questions. However, the client or significant other should feel confident that the clinician will actively seek answers to unresolved questions and problems.

15. Response to Supervision

Supervision must, by definition, concentrate on both the positive and the negative aspects of whatever is being supervised. There is no disagreement with the praise a supervisee receives for good performance. It is only the negative comment, the "constructive criticism," that creates problems. Yet, it is the modification of the weak or incorrect behaviors that improves the overall performance of the supervised activity and the skills of the clinician. The clinician should view her supervisor as her clinical teacher, not as an adversary. The supervisor's goal is to improve the supervisee's clinical performance, not to humiliate or put her down. The clinician should enter the supervisory conference as she would any learning experience. She should be open to constructive criticism and willing to discuss alternative clinical approaches with the supervisor. She should also be willing to try new strategies as suggested by the supervisor and to give them a fair evaluation while she assesses her clinical interactions. The relationship between the clinician and the supervisor should be one of teacher and student, where the focus of the interaction is to improve the clinician's clinical performance. When suggestions have been given by the supervisor, the clinician should incorporate those suggestions into the clinical interaction at the very next opportunity.

16. Informing Client/Significant Others

When parents or significant others are involved, either directly or indirectly, in the treatment program of a client, it is their right to know what is transpiring. The clinician should keep the involved parents and significant others informed about the client's progress in therapy. The information should be presented in an organized manner and without the use of professional jargon. The purpose of the interaction should be to focus on the transfer of information, not to impress the parents or significant others with the clinician's professional vocabulary. The information should be presented at an appropriate level, neither speaking over their heads nor speaking down to them. With those clients where there is need for support outside the therapy room, this need is presented to the parents or significant others in such a way as to ensure that such support will be forthcoming.

Much of this interaction may be informal, such as brief verbal reports immediately after a session regarding how well the client did that day, or ways the significant other can reinforce something that was just learned. Other interactions may be on a more formal basis, such as in a conference following a diagnostic evaluation. The appropriate balance between these informal and more formal exchanges will obviously be dependent on the situations and persons involved. It is important to keep the contacts regular and routine.

17. Interactions with Other Professionals

In almost any clinical program the clinician will find herself interacting with other professionals. She should interact with these people in a self-confident and professional way. She should speak, dress, and behave in a professional manner. She should also be aware of situations where interactions with other professionals are best initiated and carried on by the supervisor. In an academic setting, as previously mentioned, there is sometimes conflict between what is taught in the classroom and what is taught by the clinical supervisor. The supervisee should be able to tactfully and professionally handle these differences, remembering there usually is more than one appropriate method of therapy for a disorder. Ultimately, however, she is responsible to the assigned clinical supervisor as it relates to her practicum experience.

Management

18. Record Keeping

In any professional setting, it is critical that complete records be maintained on clients. This may be for insurance purposes, attendance records, legal protection, billing procedures, tracking clinical progress, or any number of other reasons. It is the responsibility of the clinician to start and maintain these records. Perhaps the most essential records are those that are kept on a session-to-session basis for each individual client. Without these records clinicians are hard pressed to remember specific details about each client, such as which techniques are being used and how well the client is doing in terms of learning a new behavior. Effective therapy is dependent on such records. The records need to be complete enough and to contain sufficient detail so that when other clinicians or supervisors read them they can do so without becoming confused by abbreviations and unprofessional jargon. The records must be written clearly and concisely and, if hand written, legibly. The clinician must follow the guidelines of the agency where she is providing service to ensure that charts, files, and other records are accurate, up-to-date, and professionally maintained.

19. Use of Stimulus Control

The stimulus, within the operant model, differs from the stimulus in a stimulus-response model. In the latter instance, when the stimulus is presented, the response occurs as a reflex reaction. In the operant model, responses originally occur without a stimulus, and their future performance is dependent on the consequence of their

NOTES

occurrence, a reward or a penalty. However, when another stimulus, such as the person administering the contingent event, becomes associated with the reward or penalty, it becomes a discriminative stimulus, which can be either positive (an S+) or negative (an S−). In these stimulus roles it prompts or cues the occurrence of the response. An S+ prompts the response to occur by signaling that the consequence for the response will be a reward. Conversely, an S− would signal the response not to occur, because the consequence for the behavioral performance will be a penalty. If there is no consequence associated with the behavior, it is extinguished and the stimulus becomes an S0.

These stimuli can be manipulated in a number of ways in order to enhance therapy. Negative stimuli can be reduced, positive stimuli can be increased, the roles the stimuli play can be changed so that an S− can be changed to an S+, and so forth. This control over and manipulation of the stimuli is essential for effective and efficient therapy. The clinician as well as the clinical environment becomes an S+ as they become associated with the rewards given in therapy. They then serve to prompt the new speech behaviors to occur in therapy. However, when the S+ are not present, as when the child is in another environment, there is nothing to cue or prompt the new speech behaviors to occur. This becomes crucial in the carry-over or generalization phase of therapy, because without the prompting stimuli the clinician must depend solely on habit strength or cognitive intervention.

Stimuli in the clinical environment will naturally assume either an S+, S−, or S0 role. These stimulus roles need to be controlled, manipulated, and used in clinical interactions to enhance the therapy. Failure to do so can impede clinical progress and negatively affect the client's incentive and motivation.

If the client is distracted from the clinical task, either in a testing or therapy situation, the clinical interaction is impeded. By controlling the stimuli, as described above, the clinician can also create an environment for her client that is conducive to learning or, in the case of a diagnostic examination, to testing. If we are to assess the client's abilities at any task, we must evaluate him under ideal conditions so that deficiencies are the result of factors such as cognitive skills or motor skills, rather than a lack of attentiveness. If therapy progress is to be charted, it is important that the therapy interactions not be interfered with by some external distraction. For these reasons the therapy and testing rooms must be arranged in such a way as not to distract from either the therapy or tests that are being administered. These stimuli are viewed as S− in that they distract the client from the clinical task at hand. So, their influence in therapy must be minimized by reducing the number of S−. Seating must be comfortable and arranged so that, if the client is expected to write or work at a table, the table is at an appropriate height. There must be sufficient light for the client to see visual stimuli and quiet enough that he can hear auditory stimuli. If the client is highly distractible, distracting objects in the room must be moved or covered up so not to distract the client from his clinical tasks. The clinician should demonstrate knowledge of the dynamics of figure–ground relationships as she prepares the therapy or test room.

20. Management of Client Behavior

If a client exhibits disruptive or manipulative behaviors in the therapy or evaluation session, clinical progress is seriously hampered. The inappropriate behaviors may be as extreme as running around the therapy room, yelling, or throwing things, or more subtle manipulation such as constantly talking about other things to keep the focus off of the difficult tasks in therapy. The question that arises here is who is in control of the therapy or diagnostic session. The clinician should establish this control very early in therapy, probably during the first clinical meeting with the client. If the clinician fails to address disturbing and distracting behaviors, clinical progress will be minimal, because therapy time is wasted in attempting to get control of the client and have him attend to the clinical tasks. It is recommended for young clients that "speech rules" be discussed during the first session to set the tone. The clinician should be familiar with the use of discipline techniques and the use of reward and penalty to manage inappropriate client behaviors. It is also important that the clinician be consistent in her application of the discipline and operant techniques. A wise clinician also recognizes when it is in the best interest of the client to seek help from the supervisor.

21. Client Motivation and Attention

Motivation is the state of need or desire within a person that activates that person to try to satisfy that need or desire. The clinician cannot directly motivate her client or his significant other, but she can manipulate important factors influencing motivation so that it is more apt to occur. These factors include such variables as interest, concern, success, and relevant reward or penalty. With these in mind the clinician can direct her therapy or conference so that the probability for motivation to occur is greatly enhanced. Without motivation clinical progress will be at a minimum. Adult clients are typically self-motivated to resolve their communication problems. Even so, the clinician cannot expect this motivation to always be present or to continue. She still must manipulate variables to assure that they are and will remain motivated. For example, activities should be of interest to the adult client, just as to a child. If an adult stroke patient has an interest in gardening, then that theme could get and maintain attention and create greater interest in the activities used to improve language skills. It is even more important to capture the interest of younger clients.

With clients of all ages, being successful in the completion of tasks is motivating. The clinician should always ensure that the client experiences success. The use of an appropriate reward/penalty system also is an important way the clinician can make sure that her client attends to the task and is motivated to perform at his very best. Because motivation is so important to successful clinical intervention, the clinician should always be aware of the motivational level of her client, and constantly manipulate circumstances to increase that level.

The younger the client, the less likely it is that the client is motivated to work on his speech. These children are in therapy because an adult decided they needed it. A cognitive approach to motivation will not be too successful here. Approach motivation can be achieved in these cases through the reward system. The child will be performing the clinical behavior in order to achieve the reward, but his motives for learning are not important. The important thing is that the child is motivated and learning to perform the clinical behavior. Motives are not always important. Think of your motives when you took some of your courses in college. Were you in class thirsting for knowledge, or were you there just to get the grade? It really does not matter. You passed the classes so learning did take place, in spite of your motives.

Procedures

22. Clinical Goals Clear to the Client

Any developmental process is enhanced if the person involved in the process knows its purpose and what it will produce. Just as we believe a supervisee should set goals for themselves with the supervisor and understand the expectations, we feel the effectiveness and efficiency of therapy can be increased if the client knows what is expected of him and where therapy is going. Therefore, the clinician should make the clinical

NOTES

goals, both long-term and short-term, known to the client. Each session should be started with a clear statement of the goals for the particular session. The clinician should also make sure the client knows what behaviors he needs to perform in order to meet those goals. Periodically throughout the session and at the end of the session, the clinician should verify that the client understands the clinical task and the goals.

One common technique used by supervisors to verify that the clinical goals are clear to the client is to enter the therapy session and ask the client, "What are you working on today?" If the clinician has appropriately emphasized the objectives and target behaviors, this question will not be too difficult for even very young clients to answer.

23. Goal-Oriented Therapy

The session goals should remain in focus throughout the clinical interaction, with all activities designed to elicit goal-related behavior. The clinician should guard against getting off track. At times the client may want to talk about other things, and it may be important for him to do so, but as soon as possible the clinician should direct attention back to the task at hand. The clinician, too, may be tempted to stray from the target learning as opportunities for learning other factors arise. She should resist the temptation and remain on target. She may decide to add a new target learning later, but this should be a carefully planned change and not a spur of the moment change. For example, if the goal is for the client to demonstrate an understanding of the prepositions *over* and *under*, and the clinician is using colored blocks in the activity, this is not the time to teach colors, because color concepts are not this session's target behaviors.

24. Use of Materials and Activities

No matter how well designed or well intended teaching materials and activities are, their effectiveness is directly related to how they are used in the learning environment. The best clinical materials can be rendered useless by inept and inappropriate use. The same material or activity may be used quite effectively by one clinician and not by another. In some cases, the same clinician may effectively use the activity with one client but not the next. Materials and activities should be a means to an end, which is the production of goal-related behaviors. We have often observed a material or activity become an end in and of itself, as the client becomes so preoccupied with "winning the game" that the target communication behaviors are forgotten.

Appropriate variation in the use of materials and activities is also important. It is extremely boring for most clients (not to mention the supervisor who is observing) to do the same thing session after session. Generalization will not likely be facilitated if the newly learned skills are never tried in different contexts or circumstances.

Simple rote drill may not be very motivating, especially for young clients. On the other hand, a highly complex game can be equally frustrating. Care must be taken to provide a balance of stimulating functional activities.

If an activity is used for a purpose for which it was never intended, its effectiveness is diminished. The clinician should not only be careful in her selection of materials and activities for her therapy, she should also be accomplished in their use.

25. Effectiveness of Instructional Techniques

There are many techniques and strategies that can be used to teach. However, their effectiveness and efficiency depend on the particular type of teaching being done and on the individual being taught. Techniques and strategies must be selected carefully to meet these criteria. Regardless of reports on the effectiveness and efficiency of a technique or strategy, if it is not used properly, it is worthless. The clinician should, in selecting techniques and strategies for her therapy, carefully select those which are applicable to her particular teaching task and the individual client's learning style. She should constantly ask herself, "Is this the most effective and efficient method of teaching this particular behavior to this particular client?"

26. Evaluating Responses

In any learning situation where an individual is attempting to substitute one behavior for another, the change cannot be accomplished unless the individual recognizes when each behavior occurs and can differentiate between them. Therefore, if a client is to substitute a new behavior for the old incorrect behavior, he must be able to recognize when each behavior occurs. So, if he is to learn, he must be taught evaluation skills by the clinician. The first requirement is that the clinician must be able to discriminate between the two behaviors correctly and consistently. If she is confused between the performances, she will not be able to teach the client to differentiate, and if the client cannot differentiate, there will be no extension of the new behavior outside the therapy environment.

An error that is frequently made by novice clinicians is accepting as correct an approximation of the target behavior because it was better, or closer to correct, than the original error pattern. In some cases, it may be appropriate to accept a less than perfect production, if that is all that can be reasonably expected from the client. In this case, however, the approximation *is* the target behavior, and must be differentiated from the old production.

It is equally important in a conference with parents or significant others to accurately interpret and evaluate the responses they give to questions or the general comments they make. This information is important when planning therapy for the client. The clinician must learn to listen carefully in interpreting and evaluating the responses by all persons involved in the treatment program, including those made by the client.

27. Time-Efficient Procedure

There are many teaching procedures, but some are more efficient than others. We might consider two procedures that are equally effective in that they accomplish the same goal. However, one procedure takes one week and the other takes one month. Since the two procedures are equal in effectiveness, we make our choice based on the efficiency of the process. If therapy is to be time-efficient, the clinician must select efficient procedures. The clinical process must be time-efficient, so that the behavior-change goal may be reached within the shortest period of time.

Appropriate pacing of therapy is also a consideration. Therapy cannot be rushed in an attempt to make the process time-efficient. This results in failure and frustration and serves to reduce the time-efficiency of the process. Neither can therapy be too slow, reducing the efficiency and boring the client to the point where he loses motivation. The timing of therapy is a crucial factor, and the clinician must be sensitive to this issue with her client.

28. Clinical Flexibility

If we are using a particular strategy to solve a problem, and we find that the strategy is not appropriate and we are not making any headway with the problem, we change to another strategy we think is better fitted to solving the problem. If the client is not making any progress in therapy, we should evaluate the procedures we are using and make changes if necessary. However, in order to do this the clinician must be perceptually involved in the therapy process. She must be aware of the changing attitudes or feelings or needs of her client. And, being aware of these factors, she must adjust her therapy to these changes in the client. If she fails to do this, effectiveness of the therapy is lost. The clinician cannot preplan her activities to meet these situations, but rather must know her client and his communication problem well enough to make in-therapy changes in the focus of her session plan. If there are major changes in the client's attitudes or feelings, there might be a need to revise the entire treatment program. It is frustrating for us as supervisors (not to mention for the client) to observe a clinician continue to apply a particular technique that is repeatedly unsuccessful. When questioned later, the supervisee tends to use either the "But I was only following the lesson plan" or the "But that's what you told me to do" excuses. The clinician must be sensitive to the client and comfortable with her own abilities in order to be flexible in her clinical approach.

It is also important to be sensitive to the needs of significant others. In giving feedback following a diagnostic or reporting progress, we must monitor their reactions to be sure we are being understood, and must adjust our approach if we are not. It might also be necessary to be flexible in the amount of support expected from a significant other. For example, in the case of one client with aphasia, her spouse had been very active in therapy. He sat in all therapy sessions and practiced faithfully with her on notebook assignments several times a day at home. The astute clinician noticed that the spouse was beginning to lose his patience more easily with his wife as he became more frustrated with the demands of her care. The notebook assignments were dropped and gradually replaced with "being together and communicating" types of assignments. The point here is that the clinician must constantly monitor the need for change and be flexible enough to make modifications to achieve the maximum benefit for the client.

29. Use of Modeling, Information, Guidance, and Feedback

The teacher's main tool in teaching any activity is the stimulus that she presents to the learner. This is that part of the learning process where she presents the new behavior along with a variety of instructions on how the learner can perform it. If we are teaching someone to swing a tennis racket we not only show them how to do it, we also tell them how to hold the racket and perhaps even guide their hand into the proper grip. If the person does not perform the swing correctly we give them some feedback: "You held your hand wrong when you swung the racket. Let me show you that again." And we then repeat the stimulus and call special attention to how to hold the hand. We adjust the stimulus to the pace of the person's learning.

In therapy we are also teaching behaviors. The clinician's stimulus in therapy is made up of modeling, information, and guidance in various combinations. She primarily uses the auditory and visual sensory channels to present her stimulus, but also is free to use the bodily sense channel with various forms of guidance. By manipulating the stimulus through assorted combinations of modeling, information, guidance, and the sensory channels involved, the clinician can make the stimulus more appropriate for the individual client. If the clinical stimulus is not appropriate for the client, therapy is not effective, because the client does not understand what is expected of him. Once the client has performed the behavior, he must have specific feedback about the correctness or incorrectness of the attempt. This reflects the opinion of the clinician. It may be interpreted as a reward or penalty, but is more closely allied with providing information about a completed behavioral performance.

30. Use of Reward and Penalty

The selection of pleasant and aversive contingent events, rewards and penalties in an operant paradigm, is a very challenging task. At best, these are selected on the "best guess" of the person making the selection. These events can only be verified as rewards and penalties according to their effects on the frequency of occurrence of the behaviors to which they are applied. The rewards and penalty selected by the clinician must be appropriate to the individual client. The reward and penalty must also be appropriate for the clinical setting, such as a university clinic, a hospital clinic, a private agency, and so forth. The reward and penalty contingency must be carefully maintained, and the schedule of presentation of rewards must be appropriate for the stage of therapy it is being applied in; for example, continuous reward for fast learning early in therapy. Because the strength and effectiveness of rewards and penalties can change rapidly, the clinician must continue to monitor their effects and, if they are no longer functioning as they should, to change to another pleasant or aversive contingent event. The clinician should also avoid satiating a client with a reward so she does not have to change rewards during therapy.

31. Client Self-Evaluation

After learning how to perform a new behavior, such as a new way of holding a tennis racket, a person must begin to use the behavior in its natural environment. In order to do this the person must learn to monitor and evaluate the behavior as it is occurring. This self-evaluation then makes it possible for the person to use the new behavior in its natural environment or to modify the old behavior when it occurs. This self-evaluation is an important behavior that must be taught in the clinical program. For new behaviors to occur outside the clinical environment, the client needs to learn how to evaluate his behavioral performance. Only after there is self-evaluation can self-correction occur. The clinician should encourage this by modeling the desired behavior and encouraging the client to imitate the model. Using a "minimal pairs" approach for correcting articulation errors is one example of a method which encourages self-evaluation. The clinician might also act puzzled, as if she does not understand, to encourage the client to correct his response and then evaluate the differences between the two. Another technique, used primarily with older clients, consists of making a video or audio tape recording of the client and then having the client evaluate the recording. When self-evaluation does occur, the clinician should reward the behavior to increase the probability that the self-evaluation behavior will occur again. The clinician's therapy plan should reflect self-evaluation as a clinical goal, and there should be methods and strategies included to teach this behavior.

32. Client Talking/Response Time

In a learning situation where behavioral rehearsal is an important part of the learning process, time must be allowed for the behavioral rehearsal to occur. The rate of learning will be directly related to the amount of time allocated for rehearsal. In order to learn a new speech behavior, the client must practice it in the clinical environment. The clinician should structure her therapy so the clinical activities elicit a maximum number of behavioral responses from the client. The clinician's talking time should be aimed primarily at providing modeling, feedback, and attempts to elicit more responses from the client. Talking time should be structured for the client, not the clinician; the client must be given ample time to respond in the clinical environment.

33. Behavioral Data Collection

In order to determine if learning is taking place and to evaluate the efficiency of the teaching methods, an instructor must establish a behavioral performance baseline, followed with either periodic or continuous data collection to compare with the baseline data. This is the most efficient way to chart learning progress. The clinician needs to develop a recording system so that she has a continuing record of both the correctness and the frequency of occurrence of the target behavior. This observation is part of the clinician's cognitions in every clinical transaction, so all that is needed is the system for recording the events. Without these data there is no way of charting progress. If the correctness of the response is not increasing the clinician should adjust her clinical stimulus, check her reward, and perhaps alter the schedule of presentation she is using. Knowing the percentages of correct responses is important since it allows her to know when the objective is too difficult, or when it has been met, so as to move on to another objective.

34. Session Goals Remain in Focus

In some clinical sessions there may be more than one objective. In this instance the clinician must not ignore one goal when she focuses therapy on the second goal. In other words, regardless of the number of clinical objectives there are in a session, the clinician must maintain some clinical attention on all clinical objectives. For example, an objective at the beginning of a session might be to increase the length of time the client maintained eye contact. Later in the session the objective may be to produce sentences with easy initiation of phonation. The clinician should not ignore the continued performance of maintaining eye contact as she concentrates on easy initiation of phonation. Rather, she should continue to reward the client for maintaining eye contact even as she is teaching vocal onset. Failure to do this severely impedes clinical progress. When she ignores the occurrence of the eye contact behavior she is extinguishing the very behavior she worked so hard to get to occur in the first part of therapy!

Diagnosis

35. Test Administration

All tests have a standard administration procedure. If the test is to be valid, it must be administered according to its protocol. The examiner should give all instructions clearly and concisely, making sure the client understands the instructions. All basals, ceilings, and thresholds should be established correctly and the tests scored or marked according to the test protocol. Tests are only as valid and reliable as the administrative procedure used to administer them. If the clinician is not familiar with the test procedure, she should check this very carefully prior to the diagnostic session. During the actual administration of the test is not the time to be frantically scanning the manual for the instructions. The scoring of tests is also extremely important, particularly because recommendations may be based on the outcome. The clinician must follow the scoring procedure according to the test protocol and should double-check all figures for accuracy and objectivity.

36. Clinical Observation Skills

Observational skills are basic to assessments of performance. Much information is gleaned from observations of the individual being assessed, and this information supplements the information from more formal assessment procedures. The clinician should be sensitive to and aware of all relevant client behaviors or behaviors of significant others. This would include not only what is said or done, but also how it was said or done. The clinician should observe carefully all of the client's behaviors in the diagnostic situation, including both those behaviors being assessed in the diagnostic session and the client's general behaviors in that situation. In many instances these observations of general behavior will provide a valuable supplement to the behavioral data collected in the formal tests, yielding a more accurate and complete diagnosis.

37. *Test Interpretation and Recommendations*

Tests of any kind are only as valuable as the way they are interpreted. If the test results are not interpreted correctly or thoroughly, the value of the diagnostic examination is lost. The clinician should take great care in interpreting the results of any tests that have been administered, because recommendations will be based on these findings. Interpretation of formal tests should include the clinician's observations of client behaviors. She needs to consider her clinical observations as she evaluates test results and makes recommendations. The clinician also needs to make the necessary and appropriate recommendations for correction of behaviors that were not formally assessed by her. For example, referral to a physician, a dentist, or a psychologist may be appropriate because of observed or reported health, dental, or emotional problems.

38. *Professional Report Writing*

Things are written so that there is a permanent record; a record that can be reviewed repeatedly over time. Professional reports may be read by a variety of persons involved with a client, including other professionals as well as significant others. A report should be written in such a way as to convey information about the client to the reader. The information is provided so others involved with the client can plan their own intervention program or work with you in resolving the client's problem. The report should be well organized, written without jargon, and grammatically correct. All information contained in the report should be pertinent to the client's problem, accurately reported, and stated clearly and concisely.

Additional Clinical Responsibilities

39. *Observes Clinical Rules*

Rules are made to preserve order. Without rules, chaos would reign. Clinic or agency rules are necessary to maintain an orderly professional operation in any clinical program. In that there are so many people involved in a clinical operation it is extremely important that guidelines (rules) are understood by all persons involved so that there is a constant flow of information, continual updating of clients' data, appointment schedules maintained, and so forth. The clinician should be familiar with all clinical rules, policies, and procedures, and should follow these guidelines in all of her professional dealings within the clinic. Such behavior indicates an acceptance of professional responsibility.

40. *Prepares for Clinical Conferences*

Teachers like to have their student read the assignments prior to the classroom contact so that the student is prepared for and can participate in the class. In the same vein, when a clinical conference is arranged, the clinician should prepare for the conference by reviewing all pertinent information about her therapy and bringing the information with her to the meeting. Her review of the information should result in clinical questions for the supervisor, as well as independent thoughts about how to improve her therapy. It is advisable for the supervisee to write these questions prior to the conference. If she is an advanced clinician she should be prepared for an indirect supervisory approach where she will enter into discussions about her therapy with her supervisor.

41. *Contributes Alternative Procedures*

In preparing for the supervisory conference the clinician should develop alternative clinical plans for semester or session goals, and the procedures to be used to

NOTES

meet those goals. She should also bring in recommendations designed to adequately meet the client's needs and enhance the treatment procedures. In all cases, the alternative clinical plans should be behaviorally oriented and based on the client's performance both in the clinical as well as outside environments.

42. Written Work is Professional

All written work, including diagnostic reports, sessions plans, special reports, and other assigned papers, should be carefully written. Sentence structure, spelling, and grammar should be given particular attention. Professional terminology should be used when appropriate, but not to the point where the report or paper for a lay person is difficult to understand. The key words for written work are clarity and neatness. All written work should follow the established guidelines and time specifications of the clinic.

43. Self-Supervision of Clinical Performance

Although this is the last of the clinical behaviors deemed essential for satisfactory clinical performance, it is perhaps the most important one. Self-supervision is essential if there is to be professional growth beyond the supervised clinical experience. The entire supervision program is focused on training the clinician to be able to supervise herself and demonstrate clinical problem solving. She should readily recognize and identify those behaviors that facilitate or interfere with clinical success. She should also plan a program for improving her clinical skills, which includes both setting forth behavioral goals and implementing a program where these goals can be achieved.

SUMMARY

These are the behaviors that will be assessed and targeted for development under the CBS system. We recommend that the supervisor and supervisee read and discuss these definitions at the beginning of the term of supervision. It is important that all persons involved in the supervision experience agree on the interpretation of these skills. This may be just an individual supervisor and her supervisee, or all supervisors and supervisees in a clinical program. This discussion and agreement sets the base for use of the CBS system. By establishing this common view of clinical behaviors, communication and learning will be enhanced throughout the supervision experience. For convenience while supervising, an abbreviated set of the descriptors will be found in Appendix C.

Chapter 7

Supervisory Goals, Tasks, and Responsibilities

Clinical supervision is a multifaceted task. The American Speech-Hearing-Language Association set forth 13 general tasks that the supervisor is responsible for. In addition, there are specific supervisory goals that need to be accomplished, such as training the supervisee to perform self-supervision. Specific tasks and responsibilities associated with supervision are presented and discussed, including such things as improving the supervisee's observation and writing skills.

SUPERVISORY TASKS: PROFESSIONAL GUIDELINES

For approximately 15 years various committees of the American Speech-Language-Hearing Association have studied and evaluated the role of the clinical supervisor in the professional training of speech, language, and hearing clinicians. A position statement, "Clinical Supervision in Speech Pathology and Audiology," reflecting this in-depth study, was issued by the association in 1985 (*Asha*, 1985). The statement covered not only the tasks and related competencies deemed necessary for effective clinical supervision, but also recommendations on the training of clinical supervisors.

The supervisory behaviors that are evaluated in the CBS system are those that are reflected in the position statement. We feel certain that all clinical supervisors are aware of these task-related behaviors, and we have included them in our Evaluation of Supervision form. However, because we are addressing both the supervisor and the supervisee in this book, we will include the 13 tasks listed in the statement. If supervisees are interested in the competencies associated with each task, we refer them to the report itself.

The following 13 tasks are felt to be basic to effective clinical teaching.

1. Establishing and maintaining an effective working relationship with the supervisee
2. Assisting the supervisee in developing goals and objectives
3. Assisting the supervisee in developing and refining assessment skills
4. Assisting the supervisee in developing and refining clinical management skills
5. Demonstrating or participating with the supervisee in the clinical process
6. Assisting the supervisee in observing and analyzing assessment and treatment sessions
7. Assisting the supervisee in the development and maintenance of clinical and supervisory records
8. Interacting with the supervisee in planning, executing and analyzing supervisory conferences
9. Assisting the supervisee in evaluation of clinical performances
10. Assisting the supervisee in developing skills of verbal reporting, writing, and editing

11. Sharing information regarding ethical, legal, regulatory, and reimbursement aspects of professional practice
12. Modeling professional conduct
13. Demonstrating research skills in the clinical or supervisory process.

With these general guidelines in mind, we will discuss the supervisor and her various responsibilities, as we view them, in her role as a clinical teacher. We view her both in her diagnostic and her clinical supervisory roles. We also view her as a speech–language pathologist or an audiologist. Finally, we view her in a number of professional environments, including training programs, hospitals, agencies, schools, or any other professional environment where supervision is an integral part of the training or service program.

SUPERVISORY GOALS

Effective and Efficient Therapy and Diagnosis

All academic and clinical experiences are directed toward creating a professional clinician whose diagnostic evaluations and therapeutic techniques are both effective and efficient. The academic information forms the foundation of these professional services in that it provides information about the theory, etiology, development, maintenance, diagnosis, and treatment of the disorders. However, this information is theoretical in nature and not experiential. The application of this knowledge in the diagnosis, remediation, or rehabilitation of a disorder is entirely another thing from learning it in the classroom. Extensive knowledge of disorder types does not in and of itself mean that an individual can effectively and efficiently diagnose, remediate, or rehabilitate a client's disorder. The individual must be taught to apply this knowledge in a clinical environment. This specialized teaching is the responsibility of the clinical supervisor. She is the only one who can lead the supervisee to appropriate application of the knowledge in a clinical setting. She accomplishes this through her clinical teaching, her supervision. Good clinicians are created by good academic instruction *and* good clinical supervision.

Clinical Insight

Although we discussed insight as it is related to foresight and hindsight in Chapter 1, we need to gain a bit more insight into what it actually means. It is one of the most important ingredients in problem solving. It is the realization of relationships that exist between various factors. It is the putting together of many bits of knowledge into a single workable unit. It is the recognition of a concept by joining together what first appeared to be unrelated facts into a logical and meaningful unit. Of greatest importance to us here is how insight is related to problem solving, which we will discuss shortly. One interesting and even amusing method of illustrating insight learning is with puns, a play on words emphasizing different meanings of words, or combinations of words that sound alike. If you look carefully in this book you may find one or two examples of this. In this context, there is humor in gaining "insight" into the double meaning of the words used. The more subtle the pun, the more difficult it is to gain insight, to determine the hidden meaning. Consider the following:

Two speech pathologists were sitting talking when a language pathologist came and joined them. She asked them what they knew about *copula*. One of the speech pathologists answered, "Isn't his first name Francis and wasn't he involved with the movie 'The Godfather'?" The second speech pathologist said, "You have it all wrong. That is Shakespeare's famous line."

There are two puns in the story. The first is a direct use of two words that sound alike but have different meanings. The second is a bit more subtle. A hint for anyone who has not solved the problem: consider the definition instead of the actual word. Remember, no one ever said puns had to be good. In fact, someone once said that puns were the lowest form of humor. Case in point! The answer to the second pun? See the end of the chapter.

Self-Supervision

Self-supervision is the ability of the clinician not only to recognize clinical problems when they arise in therapy, but also the ability to solve these problems. First the clinician must be sensitive to problems that impede the productiveness of her therapy. This awareness of clinical problems must be present at all times. The clinician cannot allow a problem to exist for several months before she suddenly recognizes it. She must be constantly assessing her therapy. It is only after she is aware of problems that she can attempt to solve them. She must consider all of the factors operating in the clinical interactions and, by carefully examining all the factors, determine if a relationship exists between them and the clinical problem she is facing. If she discovers a relationship, she will also discover how to deal with it. If the clinician cannot recognize her clinical problems and then resolve them in an orderly and logical way, she will never be able to function effectively as a professional clinician.

TEACHING SELF-SUPERVISION

Recognizing Clinical Problems

Teaching styles vary from formal presentation of information, a direct or lecture style, to an indirect style where the supervisor may refer the supervisee to reference material or direct questions to the supervisee in an attempt to indirectly lead her to correct answers or insights. We feel that both styles, and all points in between, have their place in supervision. The supervisor matches her teaching style to the particular supervisee, basing her choice of style on her appraisal of the best approach for the individual. We feel that the more direct style is more appropriate for the beginning clinician, while the indirect style should be used with the advanced or professional clinician. The teaching style used is a matter of choice by the supervisor. However, self-supervision on her part will not only indicate if the right choice was made, but will also indicate, if the choice was incorrect, what the correct style should be.

The clinician also needs to supervise herself in all aspects of the clinical process. She must recognize problems she encounters in the diagnostic process, clinical planning, interactions with others, clinical management, or clinical procedures. Let us consider each of these sources of clinical problems.

Problem Areas

Diagnostic Process

Problems encountered in the diagnostic process include not only those associated with interactions with the client, but also those related to test administration. Testing problems usually center on instructions that are not clear, test procedures that are not followed, incorrect scoring or interpretation, and giving the wrong test to the client. Test selection and administration are important factors the supervisor must deal with, and if problems arise she must carefully guide the supervisee through the problem-solving process. Again, with the exception of the selection of the diagnostic tests, the CIM model will provide direction in problem solving.

Clinical Planning

Problems in clinical planning manifest themselves in misdirected therapy. The supervisor needs to work carefully with the supervisee to make sure she understands the ultimate clinical goal with each client. If, for example, the supervisee has selected a clinical goal that cannot be achieved by the client, either within a session or in a period of time, this can only lead to frustration on the part of both the client and the clinician. Improper goals might be, for example, a goal of complete fluency for a stutterer, normal articulation for a dysarthric client, normal speech for a severely hearing-impaired adult, or normal language use for a client who has had a severe cerebral vascular accident (CVA). All treatment procedures are based on the clinical goal, and if the goal is incorrect, most aspects of treatment will also be incorrect.

Interactions: Clinical and Supervisory

If the supervisee is insensitive to her client, her supervisor, the client's significant others, and other professionals, clinical problems will arise in her therapy program. This is a difficult problem for the supervisor to deal with, because the supervisee already manifests a lack of sensitivity and awareness. This may require some counseling on the part of the supervisor, or perhaps a referral for professional counseling.

The relationship that exists between the supervisor and the supervisee is also a source of problems. If the supervisee is playing games, the supervisor must recognize the games and discourage them in the conferences. She should also be aware that her own behaviors may be at fault in the relationship with the supervisee. If she has negative feelings toward the supervisee, they may be more apparent than she realizes, and the supervisee's behaviors may be a reflection of her response to the supervisor's behaviors.

Clinical Management

Problems in this area primarily concern factors that interfere with the client's learning, such as lack of motivation and attention, disruptive behaviors, or distractions in the clinic room. The supervisor must guide the supervisee through an assessment of these factors to see if they might be contributing to problems of learning. If there is a problem in this area, the supervisee must be able to determine if it is due to lack of motivation and attention, the client's disruptive behaviors or distractions in the clinical environment. Once the source of the interference is determined, the supervisee must then be able to resolve the problem. If the problem is with motivation and attention, the supervisor might have to lead the supervisee into questioning if her therapy is boring, if her rewards are no longer effective, if the client is not feeling well, or there are other factors which could contribute to lack of motivation and attention. If the problem centers on the client's disruptive behaviors, the clinician must deal with her lack of control over the client. The possibility of external distractions interfering with learning should be dealt with by the clinician carefully examining the clinical environment for distractions.

Clinical Procedures

If the supervisee is having difficulty with procedures, any number of different problems could arise. This is a complex issue. Some of the more common problems would be for the clinician to have a problem with the client understanding the clinical goal for the session, the instructional technique selected for the client being inappropriate, the clinical stimulus being inappropriate, the procedure being too fast or too slow, and the rewards and penalties being inappropriate. There are many possible problems in this area, and the self-supervision will have to be very carefully directed. Fortunately, the CIM provides excellent guidance during the problem-solving process, pointing out not only sources of problems but also solutions to those problems.

Resolving Clinical Problems

To introduce some organizational structure to teaching problem-solving strategies, the supervisor and the supervisee should approach clinical problem solving using the CIM. Each item in the CIM provides some clues as to where a problem might exist, and suggests various solutions.

The stimulus must be appropriate for the client. This means it must be adjusted to the client's cognitive level, or intervening variables such as hearing impairment, paralysis, structural deviations, and so forth. It can be adjusted by changes in the amount, duration, and complexity of the three ingredients: modeling, information, and guidance. The stimulus can be made more or less complex, broader or narrower in scope, or designed to avoid a sensory channel that is inoperative or is distorting the input of information. If the stimulus is inappropriate, the client's response will also be inappropriate. If the clinician persists in presenting an inappropriate stimulus it only serves to frustrate the client, and all clinical progress is lost.

The clinician, in evaluating the client's response, must determine the degree of correctness of the response, if it is occurring more often, if the client is attending to therapy, and how to start the next transaction.

By determining the correctness of the client's response the clinician is verifying the appropriateness of her stimulus. If the clinical problem is that the client is not learning how to produce the correct response, more than likely the clinical stimulus is inappropriate. As we said earlier, it must be adjusted to the cognitive level of the client and to any physical intervening variables disrupting the behavior; in other words, it must be tailored to the individual client's needs.

By determining if the desired behavior is occurring more often, the clinician is verifying her reward system. If the problem is that there is no increase in behavioral occurrence, the reason may be that the reward is no longer functioning as a reward, or the timing of the presentation of the reward may be incorrect, needing to be more contingent to the behavior. The reward schedule may also have to be revised so the reward is presented more often.

When the clinician assesses the client's attention, she is, at the same time, also assessing the strength of her reward and penalty system. If the client desires more of the rewards he will have approach motivation. This results in his attending to therapy so he can perform the rewarded behavior. Conversely, if the client wants to avoid a penalty he will have avoidance motivation and will not perform the behavior that is penalized. This also results in increased attention to the clinical process; he carefully attends so that he can avoid performing the penalized behavior.

If the clinical problem appears to be that the client does not seem to be able to keep up with the pace of therapy, perhaps the clinician is not assessing the success or failure of the transactions before planning the next one. If the transaction was successful and the client learned what was expected during the transaction, the therapy can progress to the next transactional step. However, if the client did not learn during the transaction, it must be repeated, but with a modified clinical stimulus or reward. The clinician should be able to determine if the problem is the stimulus or the reward when she evaluates the client's attention. If he is attending, the reward is valid and the problem is with the stimulus. If he is not attending, the stimulus might be valid but the reward must be changed. Learning cannot occur without attending behaviors, and they are dependent on motivation.

NOTES

Weakness in planning, interactions, and management will also be reflected in the CIM. If the clinical goal is inappropriate, there will be no clinical progress, which will be noted in the clinician's evaluations of the client's responses. If there are problems with interpersonal relationships, these will be reflected in the client's motivation and attention. If there are factors interfering with the client's learning, these will be reflected in both the correctness of the response and its frequency of occurrence.

The CIM is a "road map" for the analysis of the clinical interaction to determine where problems exist. It also assists in resolving the problems by focusing the clinician's attention on that part of the CIM where the clinical problem is located.

As in the clinical situation, problems arise in the supervisory interaction. Perhaps the supervisee cannot understand what she is being told, or perhaps she is not motivated, or there may be a factor of distracting behaviors interfering with the teaching–learning interaction. Whatever supervision problem exists, the supervisor must self-supervise her interactions with her supervisee and find a solution to the problem. We suggest that the supervisor can use the SCIM (as presented and discussed in Chapter 4) in the same way the supervisee uses the CIM; as a systematic way to analyze interactions and as a problem-solving tool.

As the CIM is the guide to the analysis of the supervisee's performance in the clinical environment, the SCIM is the guide to the analysis of the supervisor's interactions with the supervisee in the conference environment. Problem solving is problem solving, regardless of who is doing it.

CLINICAL RESEARCH TRAINING

Clinical research is performed to improve the effectiveness and the efficiency of clinical procedures. It is based on reliable observations of behaviors and events. Data collection in on-going therapy is not only a means of keeping track of therapy progress, or lack thereof, but is also basic training in data collection for research. However, the reliability of the data collected is dependent on the observational skills of the clinician.

The importance of observational skills cannot be overstated. Emerick and Hatten (1974) addressed the issue of observational skills when they wrote, "Among the most crucial methods of obtaining information is *observation*. Observational skills are the product of many hours of hard work. There is no shortcut to developing these skills, and each student must practice by testing his skills against established measures of subject performance" (p. 15).

The authors then go on to describe and discuss five aspects of observation that they feel are necessary for valid data collection. These aspects are (1) the focus of the observation, (2) the depth of the observation, (3) the description of what was observed, (4) the interpretation of what was observed, and (5) the implications of the observation.

Skilled clinical observers must be trained; this is one of the most important responsibilities of the supervisor. As Emerick and Hatten suggest, the supervisor can improve the supervisee's observational skills by verifying the supervisee's observational data collection by comparing it with her own. This could be accomplished through viewing videotapes of clients and collecting data on a specific behavioral event. Supervisor and supervisee could then compare data, and even review the videotape to verify their findings.

The supervisor must introduce the supervisee to research factors such as research design, sampling, dependent and independent variables, dealing with reliability and validity, basic statistical procedures, and so forth.

There should also be some training in audio and video recording. This involves the recording of events that will be the subject of a research investigation. The supervisee must know basic recording techniques and know the role that audio fidelity plays in the recording and playback of speech samples. She needs to know that if high frequency speech sounds are recorded on inexpensive cassette recorders they will be distorted. In addition, when they are played back through small and inexpensive speakers they will be even more distorted. The proper storage of data and reproduction for data analysis is a very demanding task.

DISCUSSION OF PERTINENT PROFESSIONAL INFORMATION

Because the supervisee will someday be a professional clinician, she needs to be introduced to professional issues such as ethics, continuing education, memberships in professional organizations, private practice and business ventures, professional insurance, and so forth. Professional issues are often features in journals of professional associations, so there should be no shortage of issues to discuss with the supervisee.

DEVELOPMENT OF COMMUNICATIVE SKILLS

Because the supervisee is going to assume a professional career, she needs to be able to communicate effectively. She will not only need to talk with her clients, she will be expected to talk with parents, significant others, other clinicians, and other professionals. The supervisee needs to be able to express herself effectively, using an appropriate vocabulary and correct grammar. Her thoughts must flow together smoothly into meaningful units. She must be able to speak in front of an audience and maintain their attention and interest. She should also be able to maintain her professional speech standards when talking to figures of authority who intimidate her. The supervisee's communicative skills can be greatly enhanced if, during the conferences, the supervisor demands good speech production in their discussions and when the supervisee is verbally presenting her reports or other information.

Another important communication skill the clinician needs as a professional is writing. By requiring written reports from the supervisee, the supervisor not only can gain the information she needs from the clinician, but she can also assess her writing skills. We are referring to organization, grammar, punctuation, spelling, sentence structure, and even handwriting or typing skills. As teachers we know the problems that exist here. It would appear that writing is a skill lacking in many clinicians, both student and professional. In some instances we wonder how some of our students write home. Maybe this explains why parents are forever complaining that their children who are in college never write home, they just call collect. Some of them probably do not know how to write a letter. Each of us can think of a number of our former students who have never written to us, some because they were glad to get us out of their hair, but others because we are convinced they could not write a letter.

If there is a very severe problem with writing skills, it might be necessary to refer the student to the English department for an evaluation and recommendations for correcting this deficit. Writing skills are extremely important, because almost all clinical data transmitted between professionals or agencies are in written form.

Before making a referral though, make certain that the student understands the concept and the importance of proofreading and editing. One English professor whose students never proofread or edited the papers they handed in, attempted to impress

NOTES

them with the importance of this process by posting the following note on his door, "Author's first draft—I don't know if I should try and get through life with all of its complications and problems or if I should just do away with myself and not have to face up to all of life's troubles. Final draft—To be or not to be." Come to think of it, the final draft is also the answer to the pun presented earlier in the chapter.

Chapter 8

Self-Supervision

The most crucial skill the supervisee must learn from the supervisor is self-supervision. Without this skill there can be no further independent professional growth. The supervisee needs to improve her observational and her problem-solving skills. The CIM's role in problem solving is discussed, and several examples of problem solving at various stages of therapy are presented.

INTRODUCTION

Before we start the discussion of self-supervision let us restate our definition of the term. Basically it means that the clinician does for herself what her supervisor did for her while she was learning to be a clinician. We want to reemphasize that there are two very important skills the clinician must develop before she can provide herself with supervision. These are the skills of observation and of problem solving. Let us consider each of these as they relate to self-supervision.

OBSERVATION SKILL

By observation we mean the noticing and attending to events. Observations can be either visual or auditory in nature. We view this process, as we mentioned in the previous chapter, as a data-gathering function. The supervisor observes in order to gather data for the purpose of evaluating performance. Likewise, as the clinician observes herself, she is also gathering data to evaluate her own performance. These observations could be the reviewing of lesson plans or reports, observing her inter-actions with others and the effect she has on people, her ability to manage her clients and her clinical environment, her ability to perform necessary clinical behaviors, and other such clinical observations.

The main problems the clinician faces in observing her own clinical performance are sensitivity and objectivity. The sensitivity we are considering here is the sensitivity of the clinician to the presence of clinical problems, regardless of how subtle they are. If the clinician is not aware of a clinical problem, she cannot correct it. The clinical problems can range from major, such as an incorrect goal for a client, to less signifi-cant, such as insufficient duration of a behavioral model for a client. The clinician must be able to gather data from a variety of sources: her written plans and reports, recordings of her therapy, observations of her client in therapy, and assessment of each clinical transaction. As she gathers these data she must remain objective about negative findings and use them as a basis of problem solving. She cannot afford to be defensive with herself as she "criticizes" her own therapy. Her perceptions of her therapy must be objective at all times, and she must maintain her sensitivity to the presence of clinical problems. She is not alone; dealing with clinical problems is a fact of everyone's therapy.

PROBLEM-SOLVING SKILL

Problem solving cannot occur unless the clinician is aware of the problem and it has been carefully identified. The proficiency of the problem-solving process is dependent on the clarity of the identification of the problem. If the clinician sees the clinical problem as "The client just is not performing well," the problem is so vague that there is little chance that the problem-solving process can determine a solution. The problem must be more carefully defined, such as "The client is not performing well because he is not paying attention in therapy." Now the clinician has something to work on. The assumption is that if the client were paying closer attention, he would be able to perform better in therapy. The problem of lack of attending behaviors can now be directly addressed and a solution found. In another example the clinician states the problem as "The client cannot achieve the clinical goal." Again, this is too vague. With a little more observation and data gathering the clinician might be able to say "The client cannot achieve the clinical goal. The goal behavior is much improved, but there has been no further improvement in the past month of therapy." The clinician can now work on the supposition that perhaps the behavior has reached its limit of production due to some intervening variable and that, if the variable cannot be found or corrected, the clinical goal must be revised. The more carefully the clinician can define the clinical problem she is facing, the better her problem-solving skills will serve her.

We stress here again the importance of the CIM in the problem-solving process. Not only will this model assist the clinician in determining where the problem is (that is, which part of the transaction is creating the problem), it will also direct the clinician to the solution of the problem. Clinical problems arise in all phases of therapy: getting the new behavior to occur, habituating the new behavior, and generalizing the new behavior. Therapy cannot progress from one phase to another until each phase is completed. Therefore, problem solving is important in all phases of therapy. Let us consider some examples of problems commonly associated with each phase. As we apply the CIM in our discussion we will indicate where in the CIM we look for the solutions. Remember, the CIM represents clinical interactions only and does not replace careful evaluation of clinical planning and management.

Examples of Problem Solving by Therapy Stage

Getting the New Behavior to Occur

GENERAL PROBLEM. The young client just does not seem able to learn the new behavior I am trying to teach him. I have tried to teach the new behavior for several clinical sessions and there is no progress.

SPECIFIC PROBLEMS AND SOLUTIONS. 1. The client is not motivated; he is in therapy because his teacher referred him. He is not paying attention to the clinician and thus is not learning.

Possible Solutions: Clinician's response. Check the appropriateness of the reward (Behavior 30). If the client is not motivated to work on his speech he might be motivated to work for a meaningful reward (Behavior 21). Exciting and fun therapy could be such a reward. A highly motivated and enthusiastic clinician is also helpful here (Behavior 11).

2. The client is attending to the stimulus, but he just cannot seem to get the performance right. He is getting frustrated because he cannot get the behavioral sequencing right as he performs the task.

Possible Solutions: Clinician's stimulus. The stimulus may not be appropriate for the client (Behaviors 9 and 29). It may be too complex for his cognitive level. If the cognitive level is not a problem, the stimulus may not contain enough appropriate information for the client to translate the stimulus into the correct performance. If there is a problem of his being able to move his articulators in the appropriate sequence, perhaps there is an intervening variable of physical or neurological involvement. In that case, the behavior goal may have to be revised to a less exacting performance (Behavior 3). This situation might also call for shifting the emphasis of the clinical stimulus from modeling to physical guidance.

Habituating the New Behavior

GENERAL PROBLEM. Therapy is mired down in the habituation phase. Because the behavior is not habituating, therapy cannot progress into the generalization phase.

SPECIFIC PROBLEMS AND SOLUTIONS. 1. When the rewards are removed to test the habituation of the behavior the performance falters so it is necessary to go back to the first phase of therapy again. This happens repeatedly.

Possible Solutions: Clinician's responses. The rewards have been removed too rapidly (Behavior 30). Extinction of a behavior after removal of rewards is typical with the continuous reward schedule. The intermittent reward schedule should be used when making the transition from the first to the second phases of therapy. It might also be that the rewards used should be more social in nature, so that there is a natural carry-over from the social reward of the clinician to the natural social rewards the client will receive in his outside environment.

2. As the new behavior is introduced into more general speech contexts in this phase of therapy, the behavior falters, regardless of rewards, and it is necessary to move back into the first phase of therapy.

Possible Solutions: Clinician's cognitions. Perhaps the client was moved out of the first phase of therapy too soon (Behaviors 9 and 27) or the clinical reward has lost its value and is no longer a reward (Behavior 30). If the behavior is not stable when the client is moved into the habituation phase of therapy, the behavior could falter when introduced into a variety of contexts. If the behavior is not stable, the client should be taken back to the first phase of therapy (Behaviors 3 and 28) and the behavior stabilized before moving ahead in therapy. It is always wise to periodically verify the clinical reward to see if it is still functioning as a reward.

Generalizing the New Behavior

GENERAL PROBLEM. The new speech behavior is not occurring in the client's external environments.

SPECIFIC PROBLEMS AND SOLUTIONS. 1. There is no carry-over of the new speech behavior into the client's home environment even though the behavior is stable in the clinical environment.

Possible Solutions: Clinician's cognitions. We now deviate from the cognitions the clinician is responsible for in ongoing therapy. Our concern here is about the clinician's general cognitive involvement in the therapy process. She should recognize that the significant others in the client's life must be included in the therapy program (Behavior 8). Stimulus control is critical in this phase of therapy (Behavior 19). There must be a number of S+ in the client's external environment to cue and prompt the

NOTES

new behavior to occur in that environment. If there are no S+, generalization will be an extremely slow and drawn out process.

2. The behavior falters when it is introduced into external environments even though the client's significant others have assumed the roles of S+.

Possible Solutions: Clinician's cognitions. The client might have been moved into the generalization phase of therapy before he was ready (Behaviors 9 and 27). If the behavior was not habituated when it was introduced into external environments, it may falter, necessitating going back in therapy, perhaps even to the first phase in order to reestablish the behavior. If the performance of the behavior is influenced by emotions, it might also be that the client will need some work in the habituation phase on "desensitizing" him to speaking situations that are frightening (Behavior 19). In this instance, stimulus role shift is an important factor if the client is to be able to generalize the new behavior.

CONCLUSION

The clinician must be cognitively involved in all aspects of treatment if she is to be sensitive to clinical problems, able to define them in detail, and able to use her problem-solving procedures. This includes her involvement in diagnostic procedures, clinical planning, professional interactions, clinical interactions, and the clinical procedures in all three phases of therapy. The clinical process cannot occur properly without careful planning and cognitive involvement on the part of the clinician. There is nothing automatic about the clinical process. Each aspect of it is dependent on all other aspects. If one aspect is not planned but allowed to occur in a haphazard or chance fashion, the entire process suffers.

Regardless of the amount of planning that goes into the clinical process, problems will arise. There is no way that the clinician can plan for all possible contingencies. Therefore, if the clinical process is to function properly, problematic situations that arise must first of all be recognized as problematic and then, after careful delineation of the problem, a solution must be found. Good therapy is totally dependent on this procedure, as is the continued growth of the clinician. Self-supervision is the stuff that nurtures professional growth and effective and efficient therapy. As self-supervision becomes more proficient, there is less need for a supervisor to oversee the therapy and, hence, fewer clinical conferences. This in itself should provide the supervisee with motivation to hasten the development of self-supervision skills!

Chapter 9

The CBS System:
Operational Guidelines

The evaluation of a complex teaching interaction, such as that between the clinician and the client, requires a sensitive and comprehensive evaluative instrument. The CBS system is such an instrument. It is not a simplistic approach to supervision, nor is it a subjective and unreliable system. It is a sensitive evaluative instrument that provides detailed and reliable information on the supervisee's clinical performance to augment the supervisor's clinical teaching. This chapter introduces the operational aspect of the system. It introduces each chart and form and explains how each is used in the system. It also explains how the evaluation process evolves into a dynamic learning experience for the supervisee.

INTRODUCTION

You have now reached the chapter where we will pull all of the information in the previous chapters together. In this chapter we will suggest procedures for using the CBS system in supervision of students or practitioners in speech–language pathology and audiology, and carefully review all of the charts and forms involved.

If you are one of those people who reads the last chapter of a book first to see if you want to read the entire book, welcome. You can continue to read this chapter if you want to, but we strongly recommend that you go back to the beginning of the book. The CBS system is unique because it provides a complete system for supervision based on a theoretical model of the clinical and supervisory processes. This theoretical base is cognitive behavior therapy and the CIM, which were presented in Chapter 2. Without this theoretical framework, proper application of the system is impossible. The theoretical base provides supervisors and supervisees with a specialized clinical vocabulary and a common view of 43 clinical behaviors, which enhance communication and learning in the clinical conference. These behaviors were described in Chapter 6. If you still insist on reading this chapter first, please go back and read the first eight chapters after you have finished. Then this chapter will make sense.

DEVELOPMENT OF THE SYSTEM

Before we begin discussing the use of the system, let us discuss the development and testing of the CBS system. These occurred in five phases. The first phase, the development and initial testing of the system, occurred during the fall of 1986 at the University of Central Arkansas and Wayne State University. After making corrections in the program, the second phase of testing occurred during the first semester of 1987. In addition to Central Arkansas and Wayne State University, the system was tested by five clinical supervisors in the speech pathology training program in the

Department of Logopedics at the University of Oulu in Finland. From this testing, another series of changes was made in the system during the summer of 1987. The third phase of testing occurred in the fall of 1987. During this time, in addition to the aforementioned universities, the system was also tested at Purdue University, the University of Wichita, Memphis State University, and the University of Arkansas/Little Rock. Each test program submitted suggestions to improve the system. From this input, still further changes were made in the program in January, 1988. In the fourth phase, further testing and evaluations proceeded at Central Arkansas, Wayne State and the University of Oulu. Final testing of the system, the fifth phase, consisted of testing the system for reliability.

RELIABILITY TESTING

The reliability of the CBS system was tested using 12 clinical supervisors from the University of Arkansas/Little Rock, the University of Central Arkansas, and Wayne State University. Details of the procedures are found in Appendix B. The judges, by viewing videotape samples of therapy and referring to the Quality of Performance section of the "Key to Clinical Competency" (Appendix D) rated the performance of 19 clinical behaviors as performed by five clinicians. The samples of therapy were arranged as shown in Table 9-1.

In choosing a statistical approach to the data collected from the judging, several factors were considered. It was decided that the data from the judgings could not be pooled, because each clinician's clinical level is unique, having a different set of criteria for rating behavioral performance. Therefore, the reliability of the judges was tested on each clinical sample, which also increased the sensitivity of the test of reliability. A Pearson correlation was selected to determine the relationships between the first and second judgings. This test was to determine if the judges maintained their relative rank orders of behavioral proficiencies between judgings. The results of the Pearson correlation using a two-tailed test are shown in Table 9-2.

As can be seen by these results, the CBS system is highly reliable with the supervising judges changing their relative rank order between the first and second judging on only two of the five clinicians. The weaker correlations were associated with the judgements of the performances of one of the intermediate clinicians (clinician 5) and with the advanced clinician (clinician 3). Examination of the factors involved in these judgements indicate that perhaps the judges were having difficulty with the disorder type rather than with the clinicians' behaviors, in that both clinicians were working with clients with language disorders. This might well be a reflection of difficulty supervisors experience in the supervision of language therapy. Another artifact influencing this statistic is a restricted range of judging scores, which can depress the value of the correlation coefficient. Further investigation is needed here.

A two-tailed independent t-test was then performed to rule out the possibility of the judges demonstrating a high correlation between the first and second judgings,

TABLE 9-1. Samples of therapy

	Clinician Level	Client Age	Disorder
Clinician 1	Beginning	5	Phonology/language
Clinician 2	Intermediate	8	Phonology
Clinician 3	Advanced	68	Language
Clinician 4	Professional	43	Fluency
Clinician 5	Intermediate	9	Language

TABLE 9-2. Results of Pearson correlation using two-tailed test

Clinician	df	r	p < 0.05
1	10	0.67	S
2	10	0.86	S
3	10	0.21	NS
4	10	0.77	S
5	10	0.20	NS

as was found, but having these findings mask the fact that the judges consistently raised or lowered their scoring for the second judging. This rigorous test indicated good test-retest reliability in that, on an average, the judges did not change their scoring from the first to the second judging. The results of this test are shown in Table 9-3.

It is important to note that these high levels of reliability were achieved in spite of the fact that the judges did not have extensive information about the CBS system available; this book had not yet been completed. It is also pointed out that the judges did not receive any formal training in the use of the system to help standardize their judgments of behavioral performance. They were given a brief set of instructions regarding the procedures to be used in their judging, descriptors of the behaviors they were to evaluate, the "Key to Clinical Competency," which contained the Quality of Performance scale appropriate for each clinical level and a brief statement of clinical goals and objectives for each client they viewed.

In order to achieve even higher reliability than that reported here, we would recommend that supervision programs using the CBS system formally train supervisors in the use of the system, particularly in standardizing ratings of clinical behaviors. Once the reliability of the supervisors has been established by a program, period checks can help maintain the higher reliability.

Further development and reliability testing of the CBS system is being carried on at the University of Central Arkansas and at Wayne State University. Information regarding the development and testing can be obtained by contacting Elaine McNiece or Betty Fusilier at the University of Central Arkansas, Conway, Arkansas, 72032.

CLINICAL EVALUATION AND DEVELOPMENT

Many supervisees seem to perceive the primary responsibility of the supervisor as being evaluation for a grade, for completion of the CFY, or for a raise recommendation on the job. We trust we have convinced you that the responsibilities of the supervisor are much broader and much more complex than that. You may view an evaluation system as a means of program management, but as we describe the system we hope you change your view and see it as we do, not as a management system but

TABLE 9-3. Results of two-tailed independent *t*-test

Clinician	df	t	p < 0.05
1	11	0.59	NS
2	11	0.70	NS
3	11	0.67	NS
4	11	0.07	NS
5	11	0.35	NS

as a clinical teaching strategy. We view evaluation as a means for goal setting and positive growth. Just as we teach student clinicians to use assessment in developing goals for the client, we use our evaluation system to develop goals for both the clinician and the supervisor.

Supervisors are not the only ones to participate in evaluation. In our system, evaluation by the supervisee is equally important. Supervisors participate by evaluating individual therapy, diagnostic sessions or conferences, by evaluating the overall performance at the middle or end of a term, and by evaluating themselves. Supervisees participate by evaluating themselves to help refine their skills in problem-solving and self-supervision, and by evaluating the quality of the supervision they received.

Through the evaluation process, goals are developed that will hopefully lead to improvement of both clinical and supervisory skills, as well as improved self-supervision and independent problem solving on the part of the supervisee.

Responsibilities in Supervision

The supervision responsibilities of both the supervisor and the supervisee are shown in Figure 9-1. The end result of the supervisory process should be the development of self-supervision on the part of the clinician, as was described in Chapter 8, as well as improved self-supervision of supervision on the part of the supervisor. The equal participation by both the supervisor and supervisee is essential to the successful use of the program and to the improvement of the overall clinical process. Let us

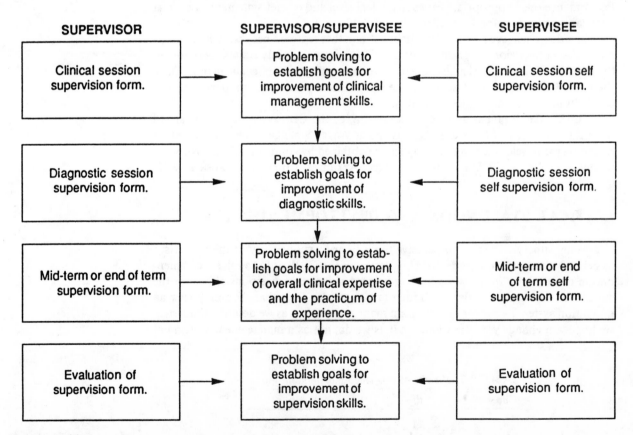

Figure 9-1. Responsibilities in Supervision. In order to accomplish the supervision goal of training the supervisee to be a competent professional clinician, able to supervise her own clinical performances, the supervisor and the supervisee must both perform specific independent tasks, as well as cooperative tasks. Clinical teaching can be successful only when these tasks are performed by both parties.

consider in general the responsibilities of both parties in supervision. Before proceeding, it might be well for you, the reader, to examine the charts and forms in Appendices C, D, and E. We will discuss these in detail later, but you should be somewhat familiar with them as we discuss the following aspects of supervision using the system.

Evaluation of the Clinical Session

Clinical sessions and conferences are evaluated by the supervisor and by the supervisee using the appropriate clinical session form. The supervisor may chose to use the form for each session observed, or may elect to rate the behaviors on an intermittent basis. The arrangements should be specified, however, so that the supervisee's expectations are consistent with what actually occurs. It has been our experience that most supervisees like frequent feedback using the form as opposed to more informal methods of feedback. The frequency for self-supervision can also be flexible. The supervisor and supervisee may agree to a schedule, such as every third or fourth session, with the option for either person to request that a self-supervision be completed and discussed more frequently. We have found that the frequency for ratings seems to be more dependent on the clinical level of the supervisee than personal preferences. The beginning clinician seems to require more frequent formal evaluation and self-supervision, with the number decreasing as the skill level of the clinician increases.

Following the independent evaluations by the supervisor and supervisee, the two should confer to compare and discuss their assessment. This problem solving may take either indirect or direct forms, again depending on personal preferences and the clinician's level of expertise. A problem-solving conference can also be held when only one of the participants has completed an evaluation. It should be understood, however, that the process of establishing goals for improvement of the supervisee's clinical management skills should be a joint endeavor. It will be difficult to effect change if the supervisee does not agree with the goals set forth by the supervisor. Targets for improvement are usually those behaviors that were rated lowest on the evaluation forms. However, in some cases priority should be given to those behaviors that might have the most positive effect on the client. The following are goals that might result from a conference concerning a clinical session.

1. Increase the amount of client response time
2. Increase use of modeling as a teaching strategy for the correct [r]
3. Improve the ability to evaluate [r] responses by spending time in the Phonetics Listening Lab listening to the [r] in various contexts.

The supervisor and supervisee will discuss strategies for achieving each goal. We recommend limiting the number of goals to from three to five so that the clinician will not be completely overwhelmed by them. Evaluation of the next session should include a specific focus on the targeted goals so that discussion of the progress toward attainment of the goals can be a part of the next conference.

This process of *evaluation-discussion-goal setting-action-evaluation* is a continuous cycle, with new goals being set when old ones are accomplished or new problems are identified.

Evaluation of the Diagnostic Session

The same process that was described above for a clinical session or conference would also be applicable to a diagnostic evaluation, either in speech–language pathology or audiology and we recommend that, whenever possible, all of a diagnostic session be directly supervised. In most cases the supervisee is not assigned to do diagnostics as often or regularly as are her therapy assignments. This means that the

NOTES

supervisor and supervisee are more likely to complete an evaluation form for each diagnostic session. Again the problem solving and goal setting conference should focus on those behaviors that received a low rating on the evaluations. Examples of goals that might result from a diagnostic conference are:

1. Improve the ability to interpret test results by writing an interpretation of examples provided by the supervisor
2. Improve the administration of a test by practicing on three subjects
3. Improve grammatical patterns and improve report writing by submitting two mock reports
4. Improve clinical observation skills by observing another diagnostic session and submitting a report of observed relevant behaviors.

Mid-Term or End of Term Evaluation

At the middle or end of the term, the supervisor and the supervisee have the opportunity to evaluate the supervisee's overall clinical performance. Their rating can then be compared and discussed in the mid-term or final conference. The second half of the supervisee's evaluation conference might best be used to suggest changes for improvement of the performance during the rest of the current term or during the next term. Such goals may be similar to ones we have mentioned previously, but also may be more general in nature:

1. Arrive 15 minutes early for all therapy sessions and on time for all conferences
2. Learn to administer three new tests
3. Prepare three new materials for use with the client.

Evaluation of Supervision

Although supervisee feedback should be encouraged throughout the practicum experience, the supervisees should be asked, at the end of the term, to evaluate each of the supervisors they have worked with. Supervisors should also be asked to rate their own performance in areas of administration, instruction, communication, interpersonal skills, professionalism, and flexibility. The rating form includes the 13 tasks of supervision previously discussed in Chapter 7. Supervisees should remain anonymous in this evaluation. This will result in a more honest evaluation. From the compiled data the supervisor should develop goals for improving her own skills. Examples of goals for supervisors are:

1. Provide more opportunities for self-appraisal by supervisees through increased videotaping of therapy sessions
2. Increase demonstration of therapeutic techniques during therapy sessions
3. Provide immediate written feedback with grades for all therapy sessions
4. Increase positive feedback in written comments and in supervisory conferences.

Supervision of Audiology

Even though using the CBS system in the supervision of audiology practicum does not differ from supervision of speech pathology, we thought perhaps we should clearly make the following statement: The 43 clinical behaviors are applicable in all therapeutic, diagnostic, or conference situations, regardless of what the specialty area is. Though the supervision of audiologists might involve more diagnostic supervision than the supervision of speech pathologists, clinical session supervision will occur during therapy with the hearing impaired. Examples of goals generated from supervision of audiometric testing or aural rehabilitation might be:

1. To improve the ability to obtain reliable thresholds with children by completing examinations on three children
2. To improve the ability to interpret impedance audiometric results by reading assigned articles on interpretation
3. To incorporate the use of the Visipitch as an instructional technique with an adult aural rehabilitation client.

DIRECTIONS FOR USING THE CBS SYSTEM

The CBS system is a teaching tool, a method of applying theoretical principles to supervison of all clinical activity in communication disorders. As a tool, it can be adjusted to meet individual needs and preferences. Do not view the system as being a rigid, unyielding method of supervision, but as a flexible means of gathering information needed for the clinical teaching process. As we discuss each of the supervision forms you should understand that each one can be used partially or entirely, periodically or continually, and singly or in conjunction with other forms. In addition, be aware that no matter what your clinical teaching style, direct or indirect, the system adapts itself to the style.

The CBS system provides a complete system for supervison: from the theoretical framework to practical application, from beginning student clinician to professional, and from observation to conference. It is, in essense, a continuum of supervision, beginning with evaluation and ending with the development of problem-solving skills and independent clinical effectiveness. The materials associated with the system are found in the appendices. They are arranged as follows:

Appendix C: Behavioral Descriptors
Appendix D: Key to Clinical Competency
Appendix E: E1—Clinical Session Supervision Form
              E2—Diagnostic Supervision Form
              E3—Clinical Session Self-Supervision Form
              E4—Diagnostic Self-Supervision Form
              E5—Mid-Term/End of Term Supervision Form
              E6—Mid-Term/End of Term Self-Supervison Form
              E7—Evaluation of Supervision Form
Appendix F: Examples of Completed Evaluation Forms

In using the CBS system, the supervisor and supervisee should first become familiar with the clinical behaviors that are expected to occur throughout the clinical experience. These are the behaviors that will be rated and targeted for growth and development. They are listed and defined briefly in Appendix C for quick reference. They are described more completely in Chapter 6. It is important that there is a mutual understanding of exactly what these behaviors consist of so there is a working clinical vocabulary to facilitate clinical teaching. The definitions we have provided serve as a guide and may be modified as seen fit. However, it is important that the supervisor and supervisee agree on what constitutes each behavior. Before the clinical experience, the supervisor should review the "Behavioral Descriptors" (Appendix C) with supervisees, either during an individual or group conference.

The next step is to determine the supervisee's expected level of clinical competency based on previous experience. The levels are

- Beginning: 0–100 clinical hours
- Intermediate: 100–200 clinical hours
- Advanced: 200+ clinical hours
- Professional: CFY and after

NOTES

This is accomplished by examining the "Key to Clinical Competency" (Appendix D) at the appropriate level. In a training program, the level is usually determined by the total number of clinical clock hours which have been completed. It is possible to make the selection of level flexible or negotiable. For example, a graduate student with 250 clinical clock hours may be placed in an external practicum site that serves a special population of clients, i.e. head injury, that she has not dealt with before. She and her supervisor may agree that it would be more appropriate to rate her at the Intermediate level, at least initially, than to use the advanced level key.

The key was developed to create different expectations for the quality of performance at each experiential level in order to prevent penalizing a clinician for lack of clinical experience. Also, because the amount of direction or supervision needed to teach a particular behavior is also a factor, the key includes the expectations for the amount of supervision at each experiential level. In rating a particular behavior, we are considering three factors: the supervisee's level of clinical experience, the quality of the behavioral performance, and the amount of supervision given to the supervisee. Thus, a good behavioral performance may be due to independent action by the supervisee, or because the supervisor spent untold hours getting the behavior to occur. The last fact needs to be considered when evaluating a behavioral performance.

With each increase in the level of clinical competency, there is an accompanying increase in the level of expectation of the quality of behavioral performance, and a decrease in the level of expectation of the amount of supervision required. This continuum of expectation is illustrated in Figure 9-2.

The top of the continuum shows the amount of supervision and the quality of performance that would be expected at the professional level, i.e. no supervisory assistance or guidance is necessary for the clinician to successfully implement the skill and demonstrate consistent independent problem solving. The lower end of the continuum shows the amount of supervision and quality of performance that would be rated "poor," even for the beginning clinician. In Appendix D, the "Key to Clinical Competency" is divided into four charts, providing expectations for the amount of supervision and quality of performance at each of the four levels of clinical experience.

With the descriptors of the clinical behaviors in mind, as well as the expected clinical competency level of the supervisee, the supervisor then selects the appropriate form for supervision. She will select either the Clinical Session Supervision form, the Diagnostic Supervision form, or the Mid-term/End of Term Supervision form.

When the supervisee performs a self-supervision of clinical performance, a review of the "Behavioral Descriptors" and the "Key to Clinical Competency" chart at the appropriate level is essential. The self-supervision, using the Clincial Session Self-supervision, Diagnostic Self-supervision, or Mid-term/End of Term Self-supervision, assists the supervisee in developing the independent clinical problem-solving skills, which are necessary for skillful therapy and professional growth.

At the end of the term, the supervisor and all of her supervisees should complete an Evaluation of Supervision form. The supervisees can provide some feedback to the supervisor on the quantity and quality of the supervision during the semester. The supervisor can then compare the supervisees' ratings of supervision with her own ratings and establish goals for improvement of supervision.

SYSTEM CHARTS AND FORMS

Behavioral Descriptors

The 43 clinical behaviors that are expected to occur sometime during the treatment program are identified and described in this chart (see Appendix C). The behaviors and their definitions are divided (as are all rating forms) into the following categories:

COMPETENCY BY LEVEL	AMOUNT OF SUPERVISION	QUALITY OF PERFORMANCE
PROFESSIONAL 5	No assistance; guidance is given by the supervisor.	Successfully demonstrates the clinical behavior creating maximal environment for therapeutic change. Consistently demonstrates independent and creative problem solving.
ADVANCED 5 4	General discussion initiated by the clinician receives supervisory approval.	Effectively implements the clinical skill / behavior. Frequently demonstrates independent and creative problem solving.
INTERMEDIATE 5 4 3	General direction is given by the supervisor at the request of the clinician.	Adequately implements the clinical skill / behavior. Beginning to demonstrate some independent and creative problem solving.
BEGINNING 5 4 3 2	General direction is initiated by the supervisor.	Displays minor technical problems with the skill / behavior which does not hinder the therapeutic process.
4 3 2 1	Minimal to maximum specific assistance / guidance is initiated by the supervisor.	Inconsistently demonstrates the clinical behavior. Exhibits awareness of need to monitor and adjust and makes changes. Modifications are generally effective.
3 2 1	Specific assistance and / or demonstration is needed with follow-up prior to the session.	The clinical skill / behavior is beginning to emerge. Efforts to modify may result in varying degrees of success.
2 1	Additional learning experience / practice / role playing is necessary. Maximum supervision is required.	Implements the skill with difficulty. Efforts to modify are generally unsuccessful.
1	Demonstration / assistance is required during the session in addition to maximum supervision prior to the session.	The clinical behavior is not evident. Makes no apparent effort to modify. Is not aware of the need to change.

Figure 9-2. Gradations of Clinical Competency and Behavioral Performance. With increased clinical experience, the supervisee's performance of clinical behaviors is expected to improve. Therefore, a behavioral performance that is acceptable for a beginning clinician may not be acceptable for a more advanced clinician. These higher levels of expectation of behavioral performance with more advanced supervisees are reflected in this figure. The five ratings of behavioral performance are shown as they relate to each clinical competency level, 5 being the most competent and 1 being the least.

NOTES

- Planning. Behaviors that occurred prior to the session as the clincian prepared for therapy, diagnostics, or conferences
- Interactions. Behaviors involved in the clinician's relationships with clients, significant others, supervisors, and other professionals
- Management. Behaviors that are related to maintaining records, manipulating the clinical environment, and managing client behavior and motivation
- Procedures. Behaviors related to the clinical process occurring during the therapy or diagnostic sessions
- Diagnosis. Behaviors that are associated with the administration and interpretation of diagnostic tests, as well as observational skills and report writing
- Additional Clinical Responsibilities. Behaviors associated with general professional responsibilities in a clinical setting.

It is recommended that the supervisor and supervisee read and discuss these definitions together at the beginning of the term or clinical experience. This may be done in a group meeting with all clinicians and supervisors or in individual conferences. It is important that all persons agree on the interpretation of the skills. This discussion sets the stage for use of the system. By establishing this common view of clincial behaviors, communication and learning will be enhanced. We recommend that each supervisee as well as each supervisor has a copy of these terms for personal reference throughout the practicum experience.

Key to Clinical Competency

This key (see Appendix D) provides a quick reference to expectations for the amount of supervision required and the quality of performance at the following four levels of clinical experience: beginning (B), intermediate (I), advanced (A), and professional (P). At each experiential level the supervisee's quality of performance and the amount of supervision required is rated as follows:

5 = very good
4 = good
3 = satisfactory
2 = less than satisfactory
1 = poor

Each of these ratings is defined both in behavioral performance and supervision requirements according to the level of experience of the supervisee; a "very good" rating at the advanced level of experience requires a higher level of performance and less supervison than the same rating at the beginning level. It is recommended that this key be discussed in a prepracticum meeting or conference so that all supervisees are familiar with the expectations for clinical skills at their level of experience. The use of this key will be further demonstrated as specific forms are described.

Clincial Session and Diagnostic Supervision Forms

These two forms (see Appendix E1, E2) are used by the supervisor to assess clinical skills demonstrated by the supervisee. Both forms have been divided into categories that refer to particular clinical behaviors that should occur prior to, during, and following the therapeutic or diagnostic sessions or clinical conference. All behaviors to be assessed are numbered and defined in the "Behavioral Descriptors." The numbers in parentheses on the evaluation forms refer to the numbers of those definitions. The clinician is rated according to the five point rating scale associated with the specific level of clinical experience on the "Key to Clinical Competency."

Using the "Key to Clinical Competency," the supervisor can rate the amount of supervision that was required in the first column (S), and the quality of performance in the second column, (P). Space is provided on the forms under each behavior for supervisory comments, and additional comments can be made on the back of the form. At the bottom of each form there is a summary evaluation/grading section for determining an objective grade for each behavioral category, as well as a grade for the overall session. The total points for supervision (S) are added to the total points for quality of performance (P) and divided by the number of scores in the (S) and (P) columns to yield an average and a unit grade. This allows the supervisor to rate only a portion of the behaviors on the forms if supervisory time is limited or if the supervisor is specifically targeting the development of particular skills. The grade may be given using the 1 to 5 rating, or expressed as a percentage, depending on the policies of the particular program or the preference of the supervisor.

In addition to evaluating therapy or diagnostic interactions, the system also provides a means of evaluating the supervisee's performance in a conference setting, regardless of the clinical mode. In order to do this, rate only those behaviors on the Clinical Session Supervision form that are preceded with a "C."

The completed supervision form should be given to the clinician following the supervision for her immediate feedback. The forms should be reviewed in the supervision conference as part of the clinical teaching and problem-solving process. Samples of completed forms are shown in Appendix F.

Clinical and Diagnostic Self-Supervision Forms

The two self-supervision forms (see Appendix E3, E4) are provided for the clinician to self-analyze specific clinical skills. These forms are used as deemed necessary by the supervisor or supervisee. Forms can be completed immediately following a session, or later using a video- or audiotape of the session. These evaluations are also based on clincial level of experience and rated in a manner similar to the forms used by the supervisor. If a self-evaluation is requested, the evaluation by the supervisor is not given to the supervisee until the self-evaluation is completed. A comparison of the ratings by the supervisor with the ratings by the supervisee may be the basis for discussion in clinical conferences. It is expected that as the supervisee develops clinical problem-solving ability, there will be increased agreement between the ratings of the supervisor and supervisee.

At the bottom of each form there is a section entitled "Goals for Development." The clinician may suggest one or two behaviors as target behaviors for growth for the next session, or the supervisor may recommend work on particular skills. In either case, the goals should be a joint decision and documented in writing. Samples of completed forms are shown in Appendix F.

Mid-Term/End of Term Supervision Form

This form (see Appendix E5) is designed to provide a summary of the supervisee's performance over an extended period of time. It includes all of the behavior competencies that have been rated in individual therapy, conferences, or diagnostic sessions, as well as additional clincial responsibilities. As with all other forms, the supervisee is rated using the 1 to 5 scales at the appropriate level of clinical experience. It is recommended that the supervisor rate the supervisee's skills as they exist at the time of the evaluation rather than an average of all individual session evaluations during the time period. The summary evaluation is scored in a manner similar to the other forms described.

This form may be completed by individual supervisors on each clinician who was supervised. If the supervisee has been supervised by more than one person during

NOTES

the term, it is possible to use the form as the format for staffing by multiple supervisors, or an average of all supervision forms may be used to determine the overall term grade.

Mid-Term/End of Term Self-Supervision Form

This form (see Appendix E6) should be given to the supervisees a few days prior to the final supervisory conferences. It should be emphasized to the supervisees that they should be honest in analyzing their strengths and weaknesses, and they should give considerable thought to proposing goals for the coming term. The supervisor may want the form returned before the conference or it may be brought to the conference. In the conference, the supervisor should review the ratings on the Mid-term/End of Term Supervision form, compare them to the ratings on the self-evaluation by the supervisee, and discuss discrepancies. This should assist the supervisee in developing her ability to self-supervise, with the ultimate goal being independent clinical problem solving. As there is a closer agreement between the self-evaluations and the ratings of the supervisor(s), the skill is beginning to develop.

The goals for development established by the supervisee should be discussed and the final conference should end with a decision regarding which skills will be targeted for improvement during the next term. Copies of all evaluation forms should be filed in the supervisee's file. However, the supervisee should retain a copy of the established goals so that the initial conference of the next term can include discussion or revision of the established goals. Just as we expect individual therapy session objectives for a client to relate to the long-term therapeutic goals, the goals established by the supervisee for development in each session should lead to achievement of the goals she wishes to complete during the term. Samples of completed forms are shown in Appendix F.

Evaluation of Supervision

This form (see Appendix E7) is designed to allow the supervisee to rate the quality of supervision received on the 13 tasks of supervision as set forth in Chapter 7. The supervisors also analyze their own perception of their performance on the supervisory tasks using the same form. Ratings are based on the following scale: 5 = very good, 4 = good, 3 = satisfactory, 2 = less than satisfactory, 1 = poor, NA = not applicable.

This form is disributed to and completed by all supervisees and supervisors during the last week of the term, but prior to the final conferences. This may help avoid a rating that is contaminated by the supervisee's grade. Supervisees' evaluations should remain anonymous. The program may designate one person such as the Clinical Director to receive the completed forms for later distribution. The evaluations are usually not given to the supervisor until all final conferences are completed. Supervisors may compare their self-evaluations to the ratings of the supervisees to outline goals for improving their supervisory skills. It is helpful to openly discuss these goals among the supervisors at the beginning of the next term.

CONCLUSION

In this chapter we have attempted to provide complete guidelines for the use of the CBS system. Because the system is very comprehensive, you may have to review the chapter several times before you feel completely comfortable applying it. As any dedicated supervisor knows, there are no simplistic approaches to good supervision. It is a complex process and it takes a complex system to analyze it. We hope the CBS system proves to be as valuable a clinical teaching tool for you as it has been for those supervisors who worked with us on developing and testing it.

References and Recommended Readings

American Speech-Language-Hearing Association (1985). Clinical supervision position statement: Clinical supervision in speech-language patholgy and audiology. *Asha, 23,* 57–60.

Anderson, J. L. (1988). *The supervisory process in speech–language pathology and audiology.* San Diego: College-Hill Press.

Block, F. (1982). The pre-conference observation system supervisors' points of view. *SUPERvision, 6,* 2–6

Brasseur, J. and Anderson, J. L. (1983). Observed differences between direct, indirect, and direct/indirect videotape supervisory conferences. *Journal of Speech and Hearing Research, 26,* 349–355.

Buckberry, E. (1982). Delayed written feedback—A supervisory approach to self-evaluation enhancement. *SUPERvision, 4,* 8–9.

Culatta, R. A. (1980). Clinical supervision: The state of the art (Part I). *Asha, 22,* 985–993.

Culatta, R. A. and Helmick, J. W. (1981). Clinical supervision: The state of the art (Part II). *Asha, 23,* 21–31.

Emerick, L. L. and Hatten, J. T. (1974). *Diagnosis and evaluation in speech pathology.* Englewood Cliffs, NJ: Prentice-Hall.

Lefrancois, G. R. (1972). *Psychological theories of human learning: Kongor's report.* Monterey, CA: Brooks/Cole.

Leith, W. R. (1984). *Handbook of clinical methods in communication disorders.* San Diego: College-Hill Press.

Lemmer, E. C. and Drake, M. L. (1983). Clinical management and professional development: A student training cycle. *Asha, 26,* 537–549.

Martin, G. and Pear, J. (1983). *Behavior modification: What it is and how to do it.* Englewood Cliffs, NJ: Prentice-Hall.

Meichenbaum, D. H. (1977). *Cognitive behavior modification: An integrative approach.* New York: Plenum.

Oratio, H. R. (1977). *Supervision in speech pathology.* Baltimore: University Park Press.

Roberts, J. E. and Naremore, R. C. (1983). An attributional model of supervisors' decision-making behavior in speech–language pathology. *Journal of Speech and Hearing Research, 26,* 537–549.

Sleight, C. C. (1984). Games people play in clinical supervision. *Asha, 26,* 27–29.

Smith, K. (1982). Critical research needs in supervision. *SUPERvision, 6,* 2–3.

Leith's Laws
of Supervision

FOR THE SUPERVISOR

1. The listening system for supervision is full of static only during those times when supervision is critical.

Corollary: This listening system will mysteriously stop working the morning of a desired supervision and will mysteriously start the next morning.

2. During important clinical observations the clinician seats the client so his back is to the mirror or video camera.

Corollary: When videotaping a clinical session for later observation, the clinician's head will be in the way so you cannot see the client.

3. Clinicans often reward their own clinical efforts in therapy by giving themselves all of the client's rewards.

Postulate: The aforementioned law is twice as valid when the rewards are chocolate.

4. The writing skills of the supervisee are inversely proportional to the length of the supervisee's reports.

5. Supervisors talk to themselves when they are figuring their income taxes and during many clinical supervisory conferences.

6. The amount of talking by the supervisee is inversely proportional to the amount of knowledge she has on the topic.

7. The choice of chocolate as a reward by clinicians is based on their glandular needs rather than on gustatory judgments.

8. The legibility of the supervisee's handwriting on her clinical reports is directly related to her performance in therapy.

9. The day you make a negative comment to another supervisor in the observation room about the client you are observing is the day the parents are also in the room observing.

10. The supervisees who need the most direction always work with those disorder types where the supervisor feels the least adequate.

Corollary: Supervisees who need constant supervision and direction always do therapy during the last period of the day.

Corollary: The student the faculty feels has the least chance to succeed in therapy is the one you are assigned to supervise in the last hour of the day.

Corollary: These are also the supervisees who miss the most therapy sessions so that substitute therapists must be found, assigned, and supervised.

11. Many clinical observations are a natural cure for insomnia.

Corollary: Clients must be survivors to come through some therapy awake.

Postulate: When the supervisor thinks she has observed the worst possible therapy, the next observation will prove her wrong.

12. The roles of clinical supervisor and mother hen are more similar than dissimilar.

13. The less a supervisee deserves a higher grade for her clinical performance the more she will protest the grade she receives.

14. Supervisees who cry about their therapy should.
15. Supervisors view life through a mirror darkly.
16. The most difficult clinicians to supervise are the ones who also belong to the debate club.
17. Old supervisors never die, they just wear away.

FOR THE SUPERVISEE

1. All clinic equipment fails to work properly when you are being observed by a supervisor.
2. The worst possible therapy sessions occur when the session is being videotaped for later evaluation.

Corollary: The best therapy sessions are neither videotaped nor supervised.

Postulate: In the videotapes of your clinical sessions you look 25 pounds heavier and 6 inches shorter than you actually are.

3. The day you decide to use the "Poor Me" game, the supervisor will play it first.
4. The day you have the conference for the mid-term evaluation is the day you wear the same dress as the supervisor.
5. The supervisors' theme song is "Do It My Way."
6. Flattery is a better supervisory game with male supervisors than female supervisors.

Corollary: Tears work better on male supervisors than on female supervisors.

7. Clinical dress codes are instigated by the worst dressed supervisors.
8. The supervisor you hear the students complaining about the most is the supervisor you are assigned to for your first clinical experience.
9. Television sets in supervisor's offices are used more for watching soaps than for clinical observation.

Testing the Reliability of the CBS System

DEFINITION OF RELIABILITY

The reported reliability of a judgment scale or other such rating instrument gives the user some idea of how stable, or consistent, the scale or instrument is over time and between judges. In other words, if a judge rates someone's performance as excellent at one period of time, would the judge rate the same performance as excellent at a later period, and how well would the judge's ratings agree with other judges? If the scale is not reliable, the judge's ratings will vary from judgment to judgment even though the performance remains constant, and there would be no agreement between the ratings of judges involved in the evaluation. The higher the reliability of the scale, the more stable and dependable it is as a rating instrument.

When we consider the reliability of a supervision system we are interested in both the consistency of the ratings by each supervisor, as well as the agreement between supervisors. It is important that the various supervisors a student clinician might work with during her training basically agree on what constitutes "good therapy," and how it is rated.

TEST PROTOCOLS

As was indicated in Chapter 9, the judgment process in the CBS supervision system is a two-factor process involving assessment of both the amount of supervision provided and the quality of behavioral performance. These judgments are basic to the evaluation of clinical sessions, diagnostic sessions, and mid-term and end of term evaluations. Because most supervision is performed on individual clinical sessions, such sessions were selected for testing the reliability of the system. It is assumed that the reliability of judges rating clinical behaviors in a clinical session would also extend to the judge's rating of other clinical behaviors in the diagnostic setting, or mid-term or end of term evaluations.

Because the judges were viewing video samples of therapy and could not make a judgment on the amount of supervision provided, they were instructed to rate only behavioral performances. Also, because the judges had no knowledge of the clinician's clinical planning, clinical interactions, and management procedures, some behaviors in these categories were eliminated from the judging form used in the testing process (see the end of this report). Those behaviors that were eliminated from the Clinical Session Supervision form were numbers 2, 8, 14, 15, 18 and 19. All procedural behaviors were included in the testing.

The judging consisted of observing the clinician's performance and determining the proficiency level of the clinical behaviors being performed. Ratings were based on the "Quality of Performance" section of the "Key to Clinical Competency," which displayed five levels of performance descriptors and associated ratings.

RELIABILITY TESTING PROCEDURES

A videotape of five samples of therapy, each 10 minutes in length, was made for testing the system's reliability. The clinical samples showed clinicans working with children, adolescents, and adults representing a variety of disorder types. The clinicians performing the therapy represented beginning, intermediate, advanced, and professional competency levels. Two of the five clinicians selected for the study were at the advanced clinical level.

A copy of the test videotape, instructions for judging, all pertinent judging information and judging forms were sent to the University of Arkansas/Little Rock (2 judges), the University of Central Arkansas (7 judges), and Wayne State University (3 judges) for the testing.

Initial testing was done at all programs in late March, 1988. Judges, seated so they had a clear view of the video screen, were given the instructions for judging, a set of behavioral descriptors of the behaviors being rated, and rating forms. After the judges had carefully read and studied the material, the test administrator answered any questions the judges had about the procedure.

When the judges indicated they were ready to view and rate the clinical samples, they were given a form containing the pertinent clinical information concerning their first observation (see sample at end of chapter). The information included:

1. The experiential level of the clinician
2. The long-range goals for the client being observed
3. The session activity objective
4. The Quality of Performance scale appropriate for the clinician's clinical level

All discussions and talking between judges or between the judges and the test administrator was prohibited from this point on in the testing process. After the judges had reviewed the clinical information and the Quality of Performance scale, the first video sample was viewed. When the sample was completed time was allowed for the judges to finish their judgments and mark the forms.

When the first judging was complete, the same procedure was followed until all judging had been completed. At the end of the judging, which took approximately one hour, the judges were requested to not discuss their reactions or judgments among themselves. The testing process was repeated approximately four weeks later and the same procedures followed.

All raw data from the judges' forms were converted into mean scores for each observation. The mean scores were used as the data bank for the Pearson correlation and the dependent *t*-test. The results of these tests were presented in Chapter 9. The results indicate that the CBS system is a highly reliable system of supervision. It is our opinion that even higher reliability than that reported here can be achieved through assigned readings and formal training of the supervisors.[1]

---

[1]For additional data on this testing, contact Dr. William R. Leith, 798 Westchester Road, Grosse Pointe Park, Michigan, 48230.

CLINICAL SESSION TEST-RETEST RELIABILTY FORM

DATE OF JUDGING: _____

JUDGING SESSION: 1 2 JUDGING SAMPLE # ___   NAME OF JUDGE: _____   PROGRAM: UCA UA/LR WSU

Rate each clinical behavior you observe as 5 = Very Good, 4 = Good, 3 = Satisfactory, 2 = Less than Satisfactory, 1 = Poor. Base your judgments on the information accompanying each video sample.

PLANNING
_____ Materials appropriate; maximum responses (4,6)

MANAGEMENT
_____ Management of client behavior (20)
_____ Client attention and motivation (21)

INTERACTIONS/CLINICAL AND SUPERVISORY
_____ Sensitivity/awareness (9)
_____ Relates to client as a person (10)
_____ Affect in therapy (11)

PROCEDURES
_____ Clinical goals clear to client (22)
_____ Goal oriented therapy (23)
_____ Use of materials and activities (24)
_____ Effectiveness of correction techniques (25)
_____ Evaluating responses (26)
_____ Time efficiency of procedure (27)
_____ Clinical flexibility (28)
_____ Use of modeling, information, guidance (29)
_____ Use of reward and penalty (30)
_____ Client self evaluation (31)
_____ Client talking/response time (32)
_____ Behavioral data collection (33)
_____ Session goals remain in focus (34)

SUMMARY—FOR STATISTICAL USE ONLY

MEAN: _____   MODE: _____   SD: _____   FREQUENCY DISTRIBUTION: 5____ 4____ 3____ 2____ 1____

RELIABILITY TAPE 1

Beth—Beginning Level—60 Clock Hours

Long Range Goals: (1) To increase imitative and spontaneous use of verbalizations, (2) to increase intelligibility by facilitating the emergence of the following phonological skills: final consonants, glides, multisyllabic productions, stridency.

Session/Activity Objective: (1) J.P. will increase spontaneous utterances to 25% of the total verbalizations (in comparison to elicited and delayed imitation), (2) J.P. will use final consonants in CVC constructions 40% of the time after modeling by the clinician.

KEY TO CLINICAL COMPETENCY
Level B(eginning)
0-100 Clinical Hours

Quality of Performance
5=Very good. Displays minor technical problems which do not hinder the therapeutic process.
4=Good. Inconsistently demonstrates the clincial behavior. Exhibits awareness of the need to monitor and adjust and makes changes. Modifications are generally effective.
3=Satisfactory. The clinical skill/behavior is beginning to emerge. Efforts to modify skill may result in varying degrees of success.
2=Less than satisfactory. Implements the behavior/skill with difficulty. Efforts to modify are generally unsuccessful.
1=Poor. The clinical behavior is not evident. Makes no apparent effort to modify. Is not aware of the need to change.

Behavioral Descriptors

PLANNING

1. *Formulates Term Goals:* Writes long-range goals for clinical behavior changes that are appropriate for disorder, severity, and cognitive level of client. Establishes priorities and gives rationale.
2. *Formulates Session(s) Objectives:* Writes session or conference objectives that are appropriate for disorder, severity, and cognitive level of client. Session objectives relate in a logical sequential way to long-term goals. Is able to separate procedures from objectives. Objectives are measurable and are written using behavioral terminology.
3. *Modifies Program When Change Is Indicated:* Recognizes the need for change when semester or daily objectives are met or deemed too difficult, and modifies therapy plan accordingly.
4. *Materials Appropriate for Client/Significant Other:* Consistently chooses attractive, motivating materials for therapy that are appropriate for client's age, disorder, and level of ability. Material for conference appropriate.
5. *Has Rationale for Clinical Procedures:* Generates procedures based on course work and outside readings. Understands and applies theoretical concepts to therapeutic and diagnostic planning.
6. *Structures Plan for Maximum Number of Responses:* Structures session plans to elicit the maximum number of goal-related behaviors by the client.
7. *Demonstration of Progress to Client:* Plans a consistent means of informing the client of gains made in target behavior performance.
8. *Significant Others Included in Therapy Plan:* Considers the influence of significant others and includes them in therapy plan. Plans for follow-up or carry-over activities.

INTERACTIONS: CLINICAL AND SUPERVISORY

9. *Sensitivity/Awareness:* Sensitive to client's needs, and adjusts accordingly. Perceptive to client's attitudes and behaviors so that circumstances can be altered to meet the underlying needs.
10. *Relates to Client/Significant Other as a Person:* Relates with respect, caring, and dignity. Priority is placed on attending to persons, not on procedures. Responds with unconditional positive regard.
11. *Affect in Therapy/Conference:* Enthusiastic and enjoys interaction. Uses language and tone that are relaxed and sincere. Interacts comfortably and enjoys working with client/significant other. Uses humor where appropriate, and is creative.
12. *Negative Personal Factors Removed from Therapy:* Keeps concerns (emotional, physical, prejudicial, etc.) from interfering with clinical responsibilities. When responsibilities cannot be met, makes necessary arrangements.

13. *Initiative/Independence:* Is able to handle case independently, and reports status to supervisor. Initiates discussion and problem solving. Takes initiative to research information related to client's disorder.
14. *Confident Image in Clinical Setting:* Displays self-confidence to parents/clients/other professionals/fellow students in the management of all disorders or clients, even when lacking related experience.
15. *Response to Supervision:* Accepts criticisms or suggestions from the supervisor(s) and constructively responds by making appropriate behavioral changes.
16. *Informing Client/Significant Others:* Relates information about client in an organized manner, using appropriate language. Addresses questions and concerns professionally. Informs significant others of the need for moral support.
17. *Interaction with Other Professionals:* Interacts in a self-confident, appropriate manner with other professionals. Is aware when interaction with other professionals must be initiated or directed by the supervisor.

MANAGEMENT

18. *Record Keeping:* The ability to follow established guidelines in maintaining accurate, professional records of client's goal-related behaviors, other pertinent behaviors, and attendance.
19. *Uses Stimulus Control:* Arranges therapy or testing room so that it is most comfortable for client and free from distractions. Uses stimulus roles for self and client's significant others to enhance therapy, particularly for carry-over. Manipulates all clinical stimuli for maximum therapeutic effectiveness.
20. *Management of Client Behavior:* Maintains appropriate behaviors during therapy and testing by setting limits and determining effective reward or penalty. Recognizes when professional assistance is necessary.
21. *Client/Significant Other Attention and Motivation:* Plans and manipulates materials, environment, and reward/penalty system so that client or his significant other maintains interest during session and exhibits approach motivation.

PROCEDURES

22. *Goals Clear to Client/Significant Other:* Presents instructions so that the client and his significant other understands the goals of the session and the behaviors needed to be performed to meet those goals.
23. *Goal-oriented Therapy:* Therapy consistently focuses on clinical goal. Procedures used are congruent with and compliment therapy goals and objectives.
24. *Use of Materials and Activities:* Uses materials effectively and efficiently in eliciting and practicing goal-related behaviors.
25. *Effectiveness of Instructional Techniques:* Uses appropriate methods and strategies to elicit target behaviors or to transmit information. Therapy and conference is both effective and efficient.
26. *Evaluating Responses:* The ability to discriminate error behavior from target behavior consistently and correctly. Carefully and accurately interprets responses of significant others during conferences.
27. *Time Efficiency of Procedure:* Appropriate pacing of therapy procedures. Therapy or conference is time efficient. Interactions are not too fast and rushed or too slow and dragging. Appropriate amount of time is spent on each activity, with smooth transitions between activities.

28. *Clinical Flexibility:* Monitoring and adjusting to client's or significant other's changing needs and performance. Recognizes change in behavior that warrants modification of program.

29. *Use of Modeling, Information, Guidance, Feedback:* Consistently uses modeling, information, guidance, and feedback appropriate for the significant other or for the age, disorder, and cognitive level of client, in the clinical interactions.

30. *Use of Reward and Penalty:* Determines an appropriate reward/penalty system for the client and clinical setting. Uses that system consistently with ongoing verification of its effectiveness.

31. *Client Self-evaluation:* Consistently models, cues, or stimulates client to self-evaluate and/or self-correct depending on client's ability.

32. *Client/Significant Other Talking/Response Time:* Structures therapy so that activities elicit the maximum number of goal-related behavioral responses from the client, with clinician's talking time held to a minimum. As client behaviors are elicited, adequate response time is allowed. Significant other allowed sufficient time to participate in conference.

33. *Behavioral Data Collection:* Determines and implements recording system. Consistently checks the correctness and frequency of occurrence of the target behavior. Makes adjustments in therapy based on these data. Progress notes indicate good qualitative and quantitative charting of behavioral responses.

34. *Session Goals Remain in Focus:* Successfully maintains focus on all daily goals throughout the session so that reward/penalty is continual and consistent. Conference remains focused on relating pertinent information to the significant other.

DIAGNOSIS

35. *Test Administration:* Test materials placed appropriately. Stimuli presented accurately and in accordance with the test manual. Basals and ceilings established correctly. Scoring completed correctly.

36. *Clinical Observation Skills:* Sensitivity to and awareness of all relevant client behaviors. Insight into the nature of those behaviors based on a familiarity with normal and disordered communication. Uses that information to support formal testing or recommendations made.

37. *Test Interpretation and Recommendations:* Describes and understands relevant communication behaviors through accurate and appropriate interpretation of formal test results. Able to determine the appropriate recommendations.

38. *Professional Report Writing:* Reports are clear, with appropriate examples or descriptions. Reports are organized, following established guidelines, and contain correct syntax, spelling, punctuation. Information in reports is accurate, concise, and pertinent.

ADDITIONAL CLINICIAN RESPONSIBILITIES

39. *Observes Clinic Rules:* Is familiar with all clinic policies and procedures and follows those rules according to specified guidelines.

40. *Prepares for Supervisory Conferences:* Brings all paperwork to meetings. Has questions and ideas for therapy, discusses impressions.

NOTES

NOTES

41. *Contributes Alternative Procedures:* Suggests alternative therapy procedures or referrals, based on client's performance.
42. *Written Work Is Professional:* Session plans, reports, and other assigned paperwork are completed accurately and neatly following established guidelines and time specifications.
43. *Self-supervision of Clinical Performance:* Recognizes and identifies behaviors that facilitate or interfere with clinical success, and develops and implements goals for improvement.

Key to Clinical Competency

LEVEL B(eginning):
0–100 clinical hours

Amount of Supervision	Quality of Performance
5 = Very good. General direction is initiated by the supervisor, or no assistance was given.	5 = Very good. Displays minor technical problems which do not hinder the therapeutic process.
4 = Good. Minimal specific assistance/guidance/direction is initiated by the supervisor.	4 = Good. Inconsistently demonstrates the clinical behavior. Exhibits awareness of the need to monitor and adjust and makes changes. Modifications are generally effective.
3 = Satisfactory. Specific assistance and/or demonstration is needed, with follow-up prior to the session.	3 = Satisfactory. The clinical skill/behavior is beginning to emerge. Efforts to modify skill may result in varying degrees of success.
2 = Less than satisfactory. Additional learning experience/practice/role-playing is necessary. Maximum supervision is required.	2 = Less than satisfactory. Implements the behavior/skill with difficulty. Efforts to modify are generally unsuccessful.
1 = Poor. Demonstration/assistance is required during the session in addition to maximum supervision prior to the session.	1 = Poor. The clinical behavior is not evident. Makes no apparent effort to modify. Is not aware of the need to change.

LEVEL I(ntermediate):
100–200 clinical hours

5 = Very good. General direction is given by the supervisor at the request of the clinician, or no assistance was given.	5 = Very good. Adequately implements the clinical skill/behavior. Beginning to demonstrate some independent and creative problem solving.
4 = Good. General direction is initiated by the supervisor.	4 = Good. Displays minor technical problems which do not hinder the therapeutic process.
3 = Satisfactory. Minimal specific assistance/guidance/direction is initiated by the supervisor.	3 = Satisfactory. Inconsistently demonstrates the clinical behavior. Exhibits awareness of the need to monitor and adjust and makes changes. Modifications are generally effective.
2 = Less than satisfactory. Specific assistance and/or demonstration is needed, with follow-up prior to the session.	2 = Less than satisfactory. The clinical skill/behavior is beginning to emerge. Efforts to modify may result in varying degree of success.
1 = Poor. Additional learning experience/practice/role playing is necessary. Maximum supervision is required.	1 = Poor. Implements the skill with difficulty. Efforts to modify are generally unsuccessful.

LEVEL A(dvanced):
200–300 clinical hours

Amount of Supervision	Quality of Performance
5 = Very good. General discussion initiated by the clinician receives supervisory approval, or no assistance was given.	5 = Very good. Effectively implements the clinical skill/behavior. Frequently demonstrates independent and creative problem solving.
4 = Good. General direction is given by the supervisor at the request of the clinician.	4 = Good. Adequately implements the clinical skill/behavior. Beginning to demonstrate some independent and creative problem solving.
3 = Satisfactory. General direction is initiated by the supervisor.	3 = Satisfactory. Displays minor technical problems which do not hinder the therapeutic process.
2 = Less than satisfactory. Minimal specific assistance/guidance/direction is initiated by the supervisor.	2 = Less than satisfactory. Inconsistently demonstrates clinical behavior/skill. Exhibits awareness of the need to monitor and adjust and make changes. Modifications are generally effective.
1 = Poor. Specific assistance and/or demonstration is needed, with follow-up prior to the session.	1 = Poor. The clinical skill/behavior is beginning to emerge. Efforts to modify may result in varying degrees of success.

LEVEL P(rofessional):
CFY/Beyond

Amount of Supervision	Quality of Performance
5 = Very good. No assistance/guidance is given by the supervisor.	5 = Very good. Successfully demonstrates the clinical behavior creating maximal environment for therapeutic change. Consistently demonstrates independent and creative problem solving.
4 = Good. General discussion initiated by the clinician receives supervisory approval.	4 = Good. Effectively implements the clinical skill/behavior. Frequently demonstrates independent and creative problem solving.
3 = Satisfactory. General direction is given by the supervisor at the request of the clinician.	3 = Satisfactory. Adequately implements the clinical skill/behavior. Beginning to demonstrate some independent and creative problem solving.
2 = Less than satisfactory. General direction is initiated by the supervisor.	2 = Less than satisfactory. Displays minor technical problems which do not hinder the therapeutic process.
1 = Poor. Minimal to maximum specific assistance/guidance/direction is initiated by the supervisor.	1 = Poor. Inconsistently demonstrates the clinical behavior. Exhibits awareness of need to monitor and adjust and makes changes. Modifications are generally effective.

CBS Supervision Forms

E1—CLINICAL SESSION SUPERVISION FORM

CLINICIAN _____ CLINICAL LEVEL* ____ CLIENT _____ DATE _____

SUPERVISOR _____ SUPERVISION OF: THERAPY SESSION ____ CONFERENCE ____ AGENCY _____

*Clinical Level: B/eginning: 0–100 HOURS; I/ntermediate: 100–200 HOURS; A/dvanced: 200–300 HOURS; P/rofessional: CFY/BEYOND

NOTE: 1. Rate only *pertinent* behaviors. Use "Key to Clinical Competencies" to rate amount of supervision (S), first column, and quality of performance (P), second column. 5 = Very good; 4 = Good; 3 = Satisfactory; 2 = Less than satisfactory; 1 = Poor.
2. Numbers in ( ) refer to the description of the particular behavior in the "Behavioral Descriptors."
3. C = Items for rating conferences; SO = significant others.

PLANNING

S   P

C____ ____ Formulates session(s) ojectives (2)

C____ ____ Materials appropriate; maximum responses (4,6)

____ ____ SO included in therapy (8)

INTERACTIONS: CLINICAL AND SUPERVISORY

S   P

____ ____ Sensitivity/awareness (9)

C____ ____ Relates to client/SO as a person (10)

C____ ____ Affect and confidence in therapy/conference (11,14)

C____ ____ Response to supervision (15)

CLINICAL MANAGEMENT

S   P

____ ____ Record keeping (18)

____ ____ Use of stimulus control (19)

____ ____ Management of client behavior (20)

C____ ____ Client/SO attention and motivation (21)

PROCEDURES

S   P

C____ ____ Goals clear to client/SO (22)

____ ____ Goal-oriented therapy (23

____ ____ Use of materials and activities (24)

C____ ____ Effectiveness of instructional techniques (25)

C____ ____ Evaluating responses (26)

C____ ____ Time efficiency of procedure (27)

C____ ____ Clinical flexibility (28)

C____ ____ Use of modeling, information, guidance, feedback (29)

____ ____ Use of reward and penalty (30)

____ ____ Client self-evaluation (31)

C____ ____ Client/SO talking/response time (32)

____ ____ Behavioral data collection (33)

C____ ____ Session goals remain in focus (34)

SUMMARY EVALUATION—GRADING   (ADDITIONAL COMMENTS—SEE BACK)

Task	Total S	Total P	# Scores	Average		Program Grade or Rating
Planning	_____ +	_____ /	_____	=	_____	_____
Interactions	_____ +	_____ /	_____	=	_____	_____
Management	_____ +	_____ /	_____	=	_____	_____
Procedures	_____ +	_____ /	_____	=	_____	_____
THERAPY SESSION	_____ +	_____ /	_____	=	_____	_____

E2—DIAGNOSTIC SESSION SUPERVISION FORM

CLINICIAN _____ CLINICAL LEVEL* ___ CLIENT _____ DATE _____

SUPERVISOR _____ AGENCY _____

*Clinical Level: B/eginning: 0–100 HOURS; I/ntermediate: 100–200 HOURS; A/dvanced: 200–300 HOURS; P/rofessional: CFY/BEYOND

NOTE: 1. Rate only *pertinent* behaviors. Use "Key to Clinical Competencies" to rate amount of supervision (S), first column, and quality of performance (P), second column. 5 = Very good; 4 = Good; 3 = Satisfactory; 2 = Less than satisfactory; 1 = Poor.
2. Numbers in ( ) refer to the description of the particular behavior in the "Behavioral Descriptors."
3. S.O. = significant others.
4. For rating conference, use Clinical Session Supervision form, "C" items.

PLANNING

S   P

____ ____ Actively participated in client chart review. Has a rationale for clinical procedures (5)

INTERACTIONS: CLINICAL AND SUPERVISORY

____ ____ Confident image in clinical setting (14)
____ ____ Informing client/significant others (16)
____ ____ Interaction with other professionals (17)

MANAGEMENT

____ ____ Use of stimulus control (19)
____ ____ Management of client behavior (20)
____ ____ Client/SO attention and motivation (21)

PROCEDURES

____ ____ Goals clear to client/SO (22)
____ ____ Use of reward and penalty (30)
____ ____ Behavioral data collection (33)
____ ____ Test administration (35)
____ Test administrated appropriately. Stimuli presented accurately and in accordance with the test procedure
____ Basals, ceilings, thresholds established correctly
____ Scoring performed correctly
____ ____ Clinical observation skills (36)
____ ____ Test interpretation and recommendations (37)
____ ____ Clinical flexibility (28)
____ ____ Professional report writing (38)
____ Report in appropriate format and with correct grammar
____ Source and reason for referral is stated
____ Background information is complete and well summarized (medical, developmental, educational, etc.)
____ Formal and informal tests/observations reported appropriately/accurately
____ Informal test results/observations reported appropriately/accurately
____ All relevant behaviors addressed during the diagnostic and clinical findings relevant to recommendations
____ Recommendations and referrals are appropriate, specific, and complete

SUMMARY EVALUATION—GRADING   (ADDITIONAL COMMENTS—SEE BACK)

Task	Total S	Total P	# Scores	Average	Program Grade or Rating
Planning	_____ +	_____ /	_____	= _____	_____
Interactions	_____ +	_____ /	_____	= _____	_____
Management	_____ +	_____ /	_____	= _____	_____
Procedures	_____ +	_____ /	_____	= _____	_____
SESSION	_____ +	_____ /	_____	= _____	_____

E3—CLINICAL SESSION SELF-SUPERVISION FORM

NAME _____ CLINICAL LEVEL* ____ DATE _____ CLIENT _____

SUPERVISOR _____ AGENCY _____
*Clinical Level: B/eginning: 0–100 HOURS; I/ntermediate: 100–200 HOURS; A/dvanced: 200–300 HOURS; P/rofessional: CFY/BEYOND

NOTE: 1. Rate only *pertinent* behaviors. Use "Key to Clinical Competencies" to rate amount of supervision (S), first column, and quality of performance (P), second column. 5 = Very good; 4 = Good; 3 = Satisfactory; 2 = Less than satisfactory; 1 = Poor.
     2. Numbers in ( ) refer to the description of the particular behavior in the "Behavioral Descriptors."
     3. C = items for rating conferences; SO = significant others.

          INTERACTIONS/MANAGEMENT
  S   P

C____ ____ Did you relate to your client/SO as a person? Did you show caring and respect? (9,10,11)

C____ ____ Did you maintain the motivation/attention of the client/SO? Was the client/SO eager or bored? Was the client distracted by things in the room? Did you utilize the stimulus roles of S+/S−? (8,19,21)

          PROCEDURES

C____ ____ Did you make the clinical goal clear for the clinical session/conference? Did you check with the client/SO to see if it was understood? Did you restate the goal periodically during the session? (22)

C____ ____ Were the majority of your clinical interactions directed toward your specific clinical goal? Did your therapy/conference become involved with behaviors other than the goal behavior? (23,34)

C____ ____ Was the goal behavior modified/understood during the session? Was the modification significant or barely perceptible? Was the change stable by the end of the session? (24,25)

C____ ____ Were behavior changes accomplished in a reasonable amount of time? Was your therapy/conference too fast and rushed (inadequate time for cognition); too slow and dragging (boring)? (27)

C____ ____ Did you adapt to your client's/SO's changing needs/performance during the session? Did you adjust according to the needs/performance of the client/SO? (28)

C____ ____ Was your clinical stimulus appropriate for the client/SO? (29)

____ ____ Were your responses appropriate for the client and the clinical setting? Were you consistent in your responses? Did you continue to verify the effectiveness of your reward/penalty? (30)

____ ____ Did you have your client monitor his own behaviors? When his monitoring was correct, was his monitoring behavior rewarded? Did your client understand the purpose of self-monitoring? (31)

C____ ____ Did you provide adequate talking/response time for your client/SO? Did you monopolize the conversation? (32)

____ ____ Did you consistently chart the correctness and frequency of occurrence of the target behavior? Did you make adjustments in your therapy based on these data? (33)

SUMMARY EVALUATION

Task	Total S	Total P	# Scores	Average	Program Grade or Rating
THERAPY SESSION	_____ +	_____ /	_____ =	_____	_____

GOALS FOR NEXT SESSION:

E4—DIAGNOSTIC SESSION SELF-SUPERVISION FORM

NAME _____ CLINICAL LEVEL* ____ DATE _____ CLIENT _____

SUPERVISOR _____ AGENCY _____
*Clinical Level: B/eginning: 0–100 HOURS; I/ntermediate: 100–200 HOURS; A/dvanced: 200–300 HOURS; P/rofessional: CFY/BEYOND

NOTE: 1. Rate only *pertinent* behaviors. Use "Key to Clinical Competencies" to rate amount of supervision (S), first column, and quality of performance (P), second column. 5 = Very good; 4 = Good; 3 = Satisfactory; 2 = Less than satisfactory; 1 = Poor.
     2. Numbers in ( ) refer to the description of the particular behavior in the "Behavioral Descriptors."
     3. SO = significant others.
     4. For rating conference, use Clinical Session Self-Supervision form, "C" items.

PLANNING

S   P

____ ____ Did you read the case history and select an appropriate test battery? (5)
____ ____ Did you meet with the diagnostic supervisor before the diagnostic and present a rationale for a selected test battery? (5)

INTERACTIONS

____ ____ Did you relate information to client/SO in an organized and professional manner? (10)
____ ____ Did you maintain a confident image with clients/SO/other professionals/fellow students during the diagnostic? (14)
____ ____ Did you interact appropriately with other professionals involved? (17)

MANAGEMENT

____ ____ Did you manipulate the clinical environment so that it was conducive to testing? Did you present the test instructions/materials appropriately? (19)
____ ____ Did you effectively deal with any behavior problems? Did you use a consistent reward/penalty system? (20)
____ ____ Did you maintain the client's attention and motivation? Did your client exhibit approach motivation? (21)

PROCEDURES

____ ____ Did you present instructions so that the client clearly understood the goals of the session? (22)
____ ____ Did you use rewards and penalties that were appropriate, consistent, verified? (30)
____ ____ Did you determine and implement an effective and accurate behavioral data collection system? (33)
____ ____ Did you administer all formal tests accurately and efficiently? (35)
____ ____ Did you demonstrate accurate clinical observation skills with sensitivity to and awareness of all relevant client behaviors? (36)
____ ____ Did you elicit and evaluate all appropriate speech/language/hearing behaviors? Did you accurately interpret test results and make all appropriate recommendations? (37)

REPORT WRITING (38)

____ ____ Did you report formal and informal test results accurately?
____ ____ Did you describe all aspects of communicative behaviors using terminology that would be clearly understood by those reading it?
____ Did you organize your report according to established guidelines?
____ Did you use correct syntax, spelling, punctuation?
____ Did you make recommendations and referrals that were appropriate, specific, and complete?
____ Did you make necessary revisions and resubmit the report on time?

OTHER DIAGNOSTIC RESPONSIBILITIES

____ ____ Were you prompt and professional in sending information to outside agencies/individuals? (42)
____ ____ Did you evalute your own diagnostic performance and set goals for your professional development? (43)

GOALS FOR DEVELOPMENT:

E5—MID-TERM/END OF TERM SUPERVISION FORM

CLINICIAN _____ CLINICAL LEVEL* ____ CLIENT _____ DATE _____

SUPERVISOR _____ AGENCY _____

*Clinical Level: B/eginning: 0–100 HOURS; I/ntermediate: 100–200 HOURS; A/dvanced: 200–300 HOURS; P/rofessional: CFY/BEYOND

NOTE: 1. Rate only *pertinent* behaviors. Use "Key to Clinical Competencies" to rate amount of supervision (S), first column, and quality of performance (P), second column. 5 = Very good; 4 = Good; 3 = Satisfactory; 2 = Less than satisfactory; 1 = Poor.
   2. Numbers in ( ) refer to the description of the particular behavior as found in the "Behavioral Descriptors."
   3. SO = significant others.

PLANNING

S   P

____ ____ (1)   Formulated term goals
____ ____ (2)   Formulated sessions(s) objectives
____ ____ (3)   Modified program when change indicated
____ ____ (4)   Materials appropriate for client/SO
____ ____ (5)   Rationale for clinical procedures
____ ____ (6)   Structured plans for maximum responses
____ ____ (7)   Demonstration of progress to client
____ ____ (8)   SO included in therapy plan

INTERACTIONS: CLINICAL AND SUPERVISORY

____ ____ (9)   Sensitivity/awareness
____ ____ (10) Related to client/SO as a person
____ ____ (11) Affect in therapy/conference
____ ____ (12) Personal factors removed form therapy
____ ____ (13) Initiative/independence
____ ____ (14) Confident image in clinical setting
____ ____ (15) Reponse to supervision
____ ____ (16) Informing parents/significant others
____ ____ (17) Interaction with other professionals

MANAGEMENT

____ ____ (18) Record keeping
____ ____ (19) Used stimulus control
____ ____ (20) Management of client behavior
____ ____ (21) Client/SO attention and motivation

PROCEDURES

S   P

____ ____ (22) Goals clear to client/SO
____ ____ (23) Goal-oriented therapy
____ ____ (24) Use of materials and activities
____ ____ (25) Effectiveness of instructional techniques
____ ____ (26) Evaluating responses
____ ____ (27) Time efficiency of procedure
____ ____ (28) Clinical flexibility
____ ____ (29) Use of modeling, information, guidance
____ ____ (30) Use of reward and penalty
____ ____ (31) Client self-evaluation
____ ____ (32) Client/SO talking/response time
____ ____ (33) Behavioral data collection
____ ____ (34) Session goals remained in focus

DIAGNOSIS

____ ____ (35) Test administration
____ ____ (36) Clinical observation skills
____ ____ (37) Test interpretation and recommendation
____ ____ (38) Professional report writing

ADDITIONAL CLINICAL RESPONSIBILITIES

____ ____ (39) Observed clinic rules
____ ____ (40) Prepared for supervisory conferences
____ ____ (41) Contributed alternative procedures
____ ____ (42) Written work was professional
____ ____ (43) Self-supervision of clinical performance

SUMMARY EVALUATION—GRADING   (ADDITIONAL COMMENTS—SEE BACK)

Task	Total S	Total P	# Scores	Average	Program Grade or Rating
Planning	_____ +	_____ /	_____	= _____	_____
Interactions	_____ +	_____ /	_____	= _____	_____
Management	_____ +	_____ /	_____	= _____	_____
Procedures	_____ +	_____ /	_____	= _____	_____
Diagnosis	_____ +	_____ /	_____	= _____	_____
Additional	_____ +	_____ /	_____	= _____	_____

FINAL GRADE $\dfrac{\text{Total score}}{\text{(\# scores)}}$ = RECOMMENDED GRADE _____

GOALS FOR DEVELOPMENT:

E6—MID-TERM/END OF TERM SELF-SUPERVISION FORM

NAME _____ CLINICAL LEVEL* ____ DATE _____ CLIENT _____

SUPERVISOR _____ AGENCY _____
*Clinical Level: B/eginning: 0–100 HOURS; I/ntermediate: 100–200 HOURS; A/dvanced: 200–300 HOURS; P/rofessional: CFY/BEYOND

NOTE: 1. Rate only *pertinent* behaviors. Use "Key to Clinical Competencies" to rate amount of supervision (S), first column, and quality of performance (P), second column. 5 = Very good; 4 = Good; 3 = Satisfactory; 2 = Less than satisfactory; 1 = Poor.
       2. Numbers in ( ) refer to the description of the particular behavior in the "Behavioral Descriptors."
       3. SO = significant others.

PLANNING

S   P

____ ____ Did you plan reasonable and appropriate semester goals and daily semester objectives? Did you research material for better understanding of the disorder? (1,5)
____ ____ Were you familiar with client's needs so you could effectively plan therapy or a conference? (2,3)
____ ____ Did you select, organize and use goal-oriented materials? Did you plan activities that were interesting and motivating? (4)
____ ____ Did you include SO in planning for therapy? (8)

INTERACTIONS: CLINICAL AND SUPERVISORY

____ ____ Did you build rapport with client/SO that was based on sensitivity, respect, and caring? (9,10)
____ ____ Were you enthusiastic and creative, and did your affect indicate that you enjoyed what you were doing? (11)
____ ____ Did you keep personal factors from interfering with clinical responsibilities? (12)
____ ____ Did you demonstrate initiative, independence, and self-confidence in your clinical management? (13,14)
____ ____ Did you build rapport with your supervisor and appropriately respond to supervision? (15)
____ ____ Did you appropriately inform clients/SO regarding clinical matters? (16)

MANAGEMENT

____ ____ Were lesson plans and progress/diagnostic reports accurate, professional, and turned in on time? Did you keep the files current? (18)
____ ____ Did you create a clinical environment that was conducive to learning or testing? Did you use stimulus control? (19)
____ ____ Did you effectively deal with any behavior problems? Did you use a consistent reward/penalty system? (20)
____ ____ Did you maintain client/SO attention and motivation? Did your client/SO exhibit approach motivation? (21)

PROCEDURES

____ ____ Were your behavioral expectations clear to your client/SO? (22)
____ ____ Was your therapy always focused on goals? Did your goals remain in focus throughout your sessions? (23,34)
____ ____ Were your materials and activities the most efficient/effective means of eliciting goal-directed behavior? (24)
____ ____ Did you use appropriate instructional techniques? (25)
____ ____ Did you discriminate errors from target behaviors, acccurately interpret reponses of SO? (26)
____ ____ Did you demonstrate appropriate pacing of therapy/conference? (27)
____ ____ Did you continuously monitor and adjust to client's/SO's changing needs and performance? (28)
____ ____ Did you use modeling, guidance, and information that was appropriate to the disorder, client, and SO? (29)
____ ____ Did you use a reward and penalty that was appropriate, consistent, verified, etc.?

DIAGNOSIS

____ ____ Did you administer all formal tests accurately and efficiently? (35)
____ ____ Did you demonstrate accurate clinical observation skills? (36)
____ ____ Did you elicit and evaluate all appropriate speech/language/hearing behaviors? Did you accurately interpret test results and make all appropriate recommendations? (37)

ADDITIONAL CLINICAL RESPONSIBILITIES

___ ___ Were you familiar with the clinic's policies and procedures, and follow the rules and guidelines? Did you take the initiative to fulfill practicum requirements? Was your attire always appropriate for professional activities? (39)

___ ___ Were you in attendance and on time for all conferences, therapy, and other called meetings? Were you prepared for each conference? Did you actively participate? (40,41)

___ ___ Did you evaluate your own clinical performance after every session? Did you set goals for your own professional development? Did you accomplish your goals? (43)

CRITIQUE OF OVERALL CLINICAL PERFORMANCE:

GOALS FOR DEVELOPMENT:

E7—EVALUATION OF SUPERVISION FORM

SUPERVISOR _____ TERM/YEAR _____ NAME (IF APPROPRIATE) _____

Please rate the quality of supervision you received on the following 13 tasks of supervision (ASHA, 1985). Base your rating on the following scale: 5 = Very good; 4 = Good; 3 = Satisfactory; 2 = Less than satisfactory; 1 = Poor; N/A = Not applicable.

TASK 1: ESTABLISHING AND MAINTAINING AN EFFECTIVE WORKING RELATIONSHIP

____ Conveyed clinical requirements
____ Appropriately confronted the supervisee for not fulfilling the clinical requirements
____ Conveyed the goals of clinical supervision
____ Applied learning principles in the supervisory process
____ Facilitated independent thinking and problem solving by the supervisee
____ Maintained an attitude of confidence in the student's clinical abilities
____ Maintained a positive attitude in helping the supervisee develop as a professional
____ Interacted objectively with the supervisee
____ Encouraged student feedback concerning the supervisory process
____ Communicated at a level consistent with the supervisee's professional development

TASK 2: ASSISTING THE SUPERVISEE IN DEVELOPING GOALS AND OBJECTIVES

____ Assisted in planning and prioritizing effective client goals and objectives
____ Assisted the supervisee in planning and prioritizing effective goals and objectives for clinical and professional growth (self-supervision)

TASK 3: ASSISTING THE SUPERVISEE IN DEVELOPING AND REFINING ASSESSMENT SKILLS

____ Shared evaluation procedures for various disorders
____ Assisted in determining a rationale for assessment procedures
____ Assisted in assimilating diagnostic findings to determine recommendations
____ Encouraged independent planning of assessment

TASK 4: ASSISTING THE SUPERVISEE IN DEVELOPING AND REFINING MANAGEMENT SKILLS

____ Stayed abreast of clinical intervention
____ Showed sufficient knowledge of the communication disorder for which supervision was provided
____ Served as a resource person in supplementing the student's theoretical knowledge
____ Provided direct suggestions for therapeutic intervention when appropriate
____ Encouraged student-initiated strategies for therapeutic intervention
____ Motivated the supervisee to develop clinical management skills

TASK 5: DEMONSTRATING OR INTERACTING WITH THE SUPERVISEE IN THE CLINICAL PROCESS

____ Demonstrated therapeutic techniques when appropriate
____ Demonstrated sufficient clinical expertise with the disorder for which supervision was provided
____ Fostered a professional partnership spirit throughout supervision

TASK 6: ASSISTING THE SUPERVISEE IN OBSERVING AND ANALYZING ASSESSMENT AND TREATMENT SESSIONS

____ Accurately recorded data derived from treatment sessions
____ Assisted the supervisee in learning and executing methods of data collection
____ Assisted in revising client treatment plans based on data obtained

TASK 7: ASSISTING THE SUPERVISEE IN THE DEVELOPMENT AND MAINTENANCE OF CLINICAL AND SUPERVISORY RECORDS

____ Assisted in applying record-keeping systems to supervisory and clinical processes
____ Assisted in organizing records to facilitate easy retrieval of information
____ Maintained the specified standards for clinical records
____ Returned paperwork promptly
____ Showed evidence of having reviewed session plans, reports, etc., when appropriate
____ Assisted the supervisee in following policies to protect confidentiality of clinical and supervisory records
____ Shared information regarding documentation for various accrediting, regulatory, and referral agencies

TASK 8: INTERACTING WITH THE SUPERVISEE IN PLANNING, EXECUTING AND ANALYZING SUPERVISORY CONFERENCES

____ Held a sufficient number of supervisory conferences
____ Allowed the supervisee sufficient opportunity to interact during the supervisory conference
____ Facilitated the supervisee's self-exploration and problem solving
____ Adjusted input based on the supervisee's level of training and experience

TASK 9: INTERACTING WITH THE SUPERVISEE IN EVALUATION OF CLINICAL PERFORMANCE

____ Identified specific clinical strengths
____ Identified specific behaviors to be modified
____ Provided immediate feedback of supervisee's clinical performance
____ Evaluated clinical performance often enough
____ Observed a sufficient number of therapy sessions
____ Demonstrated fairness in evaluating the supervisee's performance
____ Encouraged the supervisee's self-appraisal of her clinical behavior

TASK 10: ASSISTING THE SUPERVISEE IN DEVELOPING SKILLS OF VERBAL REPORTING, WRITING, AND EDITING

____ Assisted in identifying appropriate information to include in report
____ Assisted in using appropriate professional terminology and style
____ Edited reports while preserving supervisee's writing style

TASK 11: SHARING INFORMATION REGARDING ETHICAL, LEGAL, REGULATORY, AND REIMBURSEMENT ASPECTS OF THE PROFESSION

____ Communicated a knowledge of the ASHA Code of Ethics, and state licensing regulations
____ Communicated a knowledge of legal and regulatory aspects of the profession
____ Communicated a knowledge of supervisee rights and appeal process

TASK 12: MODELING PROFESSIONAL CONDUCT

____ Maintained an appropriate responsibility to the client
____ Provided an appropriate professional model
____ Met and respected deadlines
____ Demonstrated continued professional growth

TASK 13: DEMONSTRATING RESEARCH SKILLS IN THE CLINICAL OR SUPERVISORY PROCESSES

____ Interpreted and disseminated clinical or supervisory research
____ Formulated clinical or supervisory research questions
____ Tested clinical or supervisory hypotheses
____ Appropriately assigned outside readings to the supervisee

COMMENTS REGARDING SUPERVISOR'S STRENGTHS AND WEAKNESSES:

_____

_____

_____

Examples of Completed Supervision Forms

CLINICAL SESSION SUPERVISION FORM
DIAGNOSTIC SESSION SUPERVISION FORM
CLINICAL SESSION SELF-SUPERVISION FORM
DIAGNOSTIC SESSION SELF-SUPERVISION FORM
MID-TERM/END OF TERM SUPERVISION FORM
MID-TERM/END OF TERM SELF-SUPERVISION FORM

CBS CLINICAL SESSION SUPERVISION FORM

CLINICIAN __J.C.__   CLINICAL LEVEL* __A__ CLIENT __E W__   DATE __2-9-88__

SUPERVISOR __K.M.__   SUPERVISION OF: THERAPY SESSION __✓__ CONFERENCE ___ AGENCY __UCA Clinic__

*Clinical Level: B/eginning: 0–100 HOURS; I/ntermediate: 100–200 HOURS; A/dvanced: 200–300 HOURS; P/rofessional: CFY/BEYOND

NOTE: 1. Rate only *pertinent* behaviors. Use "Key to Clinical Competencies" to rate amount of supervision (S), first column, and quality of performance (P), second column. 5 = Very good; 4 = Good; 3 = Satisfactory; 2 = Less than satisfactory; 1 = Poor.
2. Numbers in ( ) refer to the description of the particular behavior in the "Behavioral Descriptors."
3. C = Items for rating conferences; SO = significant others.

PLANNING
S P
C _5_ _5_ Formulates session(s) ojectives (2)

C _5_ _5_ Materials appropriate; maximum responses (4,6)

_5_ _4_ SO included in therapy (8) *You may want to include your observer in activities*

INTERACTIONS: CLINICAL AND SUPERVISORY
S P
_4_ _4_ Sensitivity/awareness (9) *Modifications will need to be based on attention span (see 21 below)*

C _5_ _5_ Relates to client/SO as a person (10)

C _5_ _4_ Affect and confidence in therapy/conference (11,14) *Sometimes you get a little loud*

C _5_ _5_ Response to supervision (15)
☺ *Thanks for following suggestion for modeling*

CLINICAL MANAGEMENT
S P
_5_ _5_ Record keeping (18) *You have done a good job with paperwork, etc. Keep up the good work!*

_5_ _5_ Use of stimulus control (19)

_4_ _3_ Management of client behavior (20)

C _4_ _4_ Client/SO attention and motivation (21)

PROCEDURES
S P
C _4_ _4_ Goals clear to client/SO (22) *Not always sure she knows what you want.*

_4_ _5_ Goal-oriented therapy (23

_5_ _4_ Use of materials and activities (24) *Have them ready to go!*

C _4_ _4_ Effectiveness of instructional techniques (25) *Be sure to have repetition in your repetoire of techniques*

C _3_ _3_ Evaluating responses (26) *Use the multidimensional scoring system we discussed in seminar*

C _4_ _4_ Time efficiency of procedure (27) *Pacing was sometimes a bit slow. We'll discuss in conf.*

C _5_ _5_ Clinical flexibility (28)

C _5_ _4_ Use of modeling, information, guidance, feedback (29) *You need to model more. Be more specific.*

_4_ _3_ Use of reward and penalty (30) *You're improving here*

_5_ _5_ Client self-evaluation (31) *Good job getting her to self-evaluate.*

C _4_ _4_ Client/SO talking/response time (32)

_4_ _4_ Behavioral data collection (33) *Be sure you are tracking responses carefully.*

C _4_ _4_ Session goals remain in focus (34)

SUMMARY EVALUATION—GRADING   (ADDITIONAL COMMENTS—SEE BACK)

Task	Total S	Total P	# Items	Average	Program Grade or Rating
Planning	15	+ 14	/ 6	= 4.83	96 % A
Interactions	19	+ 18	/ 8	= 4.63	92 % A-
Management	18	+ 17	/ 8	= 4.38	87% B
Procedures	55	+ 53	/ 26	= 4.15	83% B
THERAPY SESSION	107	+ 102	/ 48	= 4.35	87% B

CBS DIAGNOSTIC SUPERVISION FORM

CLINICIAN **M. K.**   CLINICAL LEVEL* **I** CLIENT **S. S.**   DATE **3-8-88**

SUPERVISOR **B. F.**   AGENCY **UCA - Audiology**

*Clinical Level: B/eginning: 0–100 HOURS; I/ntermediate: 100–200 HOURS; A/dvanced: 200–300 HOURS; P/rofessional: CFY/BEYOND

NOTE: 1. Rate only *pertinent* behaviors. Use "Key to Clinical Competencies" to rate amount of supervision (S), first column, and quality of performance (P), second column. 5 = Very good; 4 = Good; 3 = Satisfactory; 2 = Less than satisfactory; 1 = Poor.
    2. Numbers in ( ) refer to the description of the particular behavior in the "Behavioral Descriptors."
    3. S.O. = significant others.
    4. For rating conference, use Clinical Session Supervision form, "C" items.

PLANNING

S   P

3   **4**   Actively participated in client chart review. Has a rationale for clinical procedures (5)

INTERACTIONS: CLINICAL AND SUPERVISORY

4   **3**   Confident image in clinical setting (14)   *I'm sure you'll become more confident*
4   **4**   Informing client/significant others (16)   *as you gain experience.*
4   **4**   Interaction with other professionals (17)

MANAGEMENT

5   **5**   Use of stimulus control (19)
5   **5**   Management of client behavior (20)
5   **5**   Client/SO attention and motivation (21)   *Nice job*

PROCEDURES

5   **5**   Goals clear to client/SO (22)
5   **4**   Use of reward and penalty (30)
4   **3**   Behavioral data collection (33) *Your observation skills are good, but you must record what you see.*
2   **4**   Test administration (35) *You must have practiced since last time! Nice job.*
    4   Test administrated appropriately. Stimuli presented accurately and in accordance with the test procedure
    4   Basals, ceilings, thresholds established correctly
    4   Scoring performed correctly
5   **5**   Clinical observation skills (36) *Good*
3   **3**   Test interpretation and recommendations (37) *Reread the articles on impedence testing.*
5   **4**   Clinical flexibility (28)
2   **4**   Professional report writing (38) *Much improved! Our practice paid off!*
    4   Report in appropriate format and with correct grammar
    5   Source and reason for referral is stated
    4   Background information is complete and well summarized (medical, developmental, educational, etc.)
    4   Formal and informal tests/observations reported appropriately/accurately
    4   Informal test results/observations reported appropriately/accurately
    4   All relevant behaviors addressed during the diagnostic and clinical findings relevant to recommendations
    3   Recommendations and referrals are appropriate, specific, and complete

SUMMARY EVALUATION—GRADING   (ADDITIONAL COMMENTS—SEE BACK)

Task	Total S		Total P	/	# Items	=	Average		Program Grade or Rating
Planning	3	+	4	/	2	=	3.5		70% C−
Interactions	12	+	11	/	6	=	3.83		77% C+
Management	15	+	15	/	6	=	5.00		100% A
Procedures	31	+	72	/	26	=	3.96		79% C+
SESSION	61	+	102	/	40	=	4.08		81% B−

CLINICAL SESSION SELF-SUPERVISION FORM

NAME __M. M.__ CLINICAL LEVEL* __B__ DATE __3-11-88__ CLIENT __S. K.__

SUPERVISOR __S. D.__ AGENCY __CHDC__

*Clinical Level: B/eginning: 0–100 HOURS; I/ntermediate: 100–200 HOURS; A/dvanced: 200–300 HOURS; P/rofessional: CFY/BEYOND

NOTE: 1. Rate only *pertinent* behaviors. Use "Key to Clinical Competencies" to rate amount of supervision (S), first column, and quality of performance (P), second column. 5 = Very good; 4 = Good; 3 = Satisfactory; 2 = Less than satisfactory; 1 = Poor.
   2. Numbers in ( ) refer to the description of the particular behavior in the "Behavioral Descriptors."
   3. C = items for rating conferences; SO = significant others.

INTERACTIONS/MANAGEMENT

S   P

C _5_ _5_ Did you relate to your client/SO as a person? Did you show caring and respect? (9,10,11)

C _4_ _4_ Did you maintain the motivation/attention of the client/SO? Was the client/SO eager or bored? Was the client distracted by things in the room? Did you utilize the stimulus roles of S+/S−? (8,19,21)

PROCEDURES

C _4_ _4_ Did you make the clinical goal clear for the clinical session/conference? Did you check with the client/SO to see if it was understood? Did you restate the goal periodically during the session? (22)

C _4_ _4_ Were the majority of your clinical interactions directed toward your specific clinical goal? Did your therapy/conference become involved with behaviors other than the goal behavior? (23,34)

C _3_ _4_ Was the goal behavior modified/understood during the session? Was the modification significant or barely perceptable? Was the change stable by the end of the session? (24,25)

C _3_ _3_ Were behavior changes accomplished in a reasonable amount of time? Was your therapy/conference too fast and rushed (inadequate time for cognition); (too slow and dragging (boring)? (27)

C _5_ _5_ Did you adapt to your client's/SO's changing needs/performance during the session? Did you adjust according to the needs/performance of the client/SO? (28)

C _5_ _5_ Was your clinical stimulus appropriate for the client/SO? (29)

_4_ _4_ Were your responses appropriate for the client and the clinical setting? Were you consistent in your responses? Did you continue to verify the effectiveness of your reward/penalty? (30)

_3_ _3_ Did you have your client monitor his own behaviors? When his monitoring was correct, was his monitoring behavior rewarded? Did your client understand the purpose of self-monitoring? (31)

C _4_ _3_ Did you provide adequate talking/response time for your client/SO? Did you monopolize the conversation? (32)

_3_ _3_ Did you consistently chart the correctness and frequency of occurrence of the target behavior? Did you make adjustments in your therapy based on these data? (33)

SUMMARY EVALUATION

Task	Total S	Total P	# Items	Average	Program Grade or Rating
THERAPY SESSION	_47_ +	_47_ /	_24_ =	_3.92_	_78%_

GOALS FOR NEXT SESSION:

1. Use multidimensional scoring.
2. Have S.K. self evaluate more frequently.
3. Speed things up a bit and make sure transitions between activities are quick.

DIAGNOSTIC SESSION SELF-SUPERVISION FORM

NAME _J.P._ CLINICAL LEVEL* _P_ DATE _3-9-88_ CLIENT _T.J._

SUPERVISOR _B.L._ AGENCY _B. Med. Ctr._

*Clinical Level: B/eginning: 0–100 HOURS; I/ntermediate: 100–200 HOURS; A/dvanced: 200–300 HOURS; P/rofessional: CFY/BEYOND

NOTE: 1. Rate only *pertinent* behaviors. Use "Key to Clinical Competencies" to rate amount of supervision (S), first column, and quality of performance (P), second column. 5 = Very good; 4 = Good; 3 = Satisfactory; 2 = Less than satisfactory; 1 = Poor.
2. Numbers in ( ) refer to the description of the particular behavior in the "Behavioral Descriptors."
3. SO = significant others.

PLANNING

S P

5 4 Did you read the case history and select an appropriate test battery? (5)
5 5 Did you meet with the diagnostic supervisor before the diagnostic and present a rationale for a selected test battery? (5)

INTERACTIONS

5 3 Did you relate information to client/SO in an organized and professional manner? (10)
5 4 Did you maintain a confident image with clients/SO/other professionals/fellow students during the diagnostic? (14)
5 4 Did you interact appropriately with other professionals involved? (17)

MANAGEMENT

Thanks for the help!

5 5 Did you manipulate the clinical environment so that it was conducive to testing? Did you present the test instructions/materials appropriately? (19)
3 4 Did you effectively deal with any behavior problems? Did you use a consistent reward/penalty system? (20)
3 4 Did you maintain the client's attention and motivation? Did your client exhibit approach motivation? (21)

PROCEDURES

5 5 Did you present instructions so that the client clearly understood the goals of the session? (22)
5 4 Did you use rewards and penalties that were appropriate, consistent, verified? (30)
5 4 Did you determine and implement an effective and accurate behavioral data collection system? (33)
5 5 Did you administer all formal tests accurately and efficiently? (35)
5 5 Did you demonstrate accurate clinical observation skills with sensitivity to and awareness of all relevant client behaviors? (36)
5 5 Did you elicit and evaluate all appropriate speech/language/hearing behaviors? Did you accurately interpret test results and make all appropriate recommendations? (37)

REPORT WRITING (38)

5 4 Did you report formal and informal test results accurately?
5 4 Did you describe all aspects of communicative behaviors using terminology that would be clearly understood by those reading it?
   4 Did you organize your report according to established guidelines?
   4 Did you use correct syntax, spelling, punctuation?
   4 Did you make recommendations and referrals that were appropriate, specific, and complete?
   4 Did you make necessary revisions and resubmit the report on time?

OTHER DIAGNOSTIC RESPONSIBILITIES

5 5 Were you prompt and professional in sending information to outside agencies/individuals? (42)
5 5 Did you evaluate your own diagnostic performance and set goals for your professional development? (43)

GOALS FOR DEVELOPMENT:
1. Continue to focus on improving client motivation.
2. Improve ability to manipulate reward/penalty system to manage behaviors.
3. Practice report writing using BMC protocol.

CBS END OF TERM SUPERVISION FORM

CLINICIAN **M.C.**   CLINICAL LEVEL* **B** CLIENT **RG/BB**   DATE **5-10-88**

SUPERVISOR **McDaniel**   AGENCY **UCA Clinic**

*Clinical Level: B/eginning: 0–100 HOURS; I/ntermediate: 100–200 HOURS; A/dvanced: 200–300 HOURS; P/rofessional: CFY/BEYOND

NOTE: 1. Rate only *pertinent* behaviors. Use "Key to Clinical Competencies" to rate amount of supervision (S), first column, and quality of performance (P), second column. 5 = Very good; 4 = Good; 3 = Satisfactory; 2 = Less than satisfactory; 1 = Poor.

      2. Numbers in ( ) refer to the description of the particular behavior as found in the "Behavioral Descriptors."

      3. SO = significant others.

PLANNING

S	P		
N/A		(1)	Formulated term goals
4	4	(2)	Formulated sessions(s) objectives
4	4	(3)	Modified program when change indicated
4	4	(4)	Materials appropriate for client/SO
4	4	(5)	Rationale for clinical procedures
5	5	(6)	Structured plans for maximum responses
4	4	(7)	Demonstration of progress to client
N/A		(8)	SO included in therapy plan

INTERACTIONS: CLINICAL AND SUPERVISORY

S	P		
5	5	(9)	Sensitivity/awareness
5	5	(10)	Related to client/SO as a person
5	5	(11)	Affect in therapy/conference
5	5	(12)	Personal factors removed form therapy
4	4	(13)	Initiative/independence
5	5	(14)	Confident image in clinical setting
5	5	(15)	Reponse to supervision
N/A		(16)	Informing parents/significant others
5	5	(17)	Interaction with other professionals

MANAGEMENT

S	P		
5	5	(18)	Record keeping
4	4	(19)	Used stimulus control
5	5	(20)	Management of client behavior
5	5	(21)	Client/SO attention and motivation

PROCEDURES

S	P		
4	4	(22)	Goals clear to client/SO
5	5	(23)	Goal-oriented therapy
5	5	(24)	Use of materials and activities
4	4	(25)	Effectiveness of instructional techniques
4	4	(26)	Evaluating responses
4	4	(27)	Time efficiency of procedure
5	5	(28)	Clinical flexibility
4	4	(29)	Use of modeling, information, guidance
4	4	(30)	Use of reward and penalty
5	5	(31)	Client self-evaluation
5	5	(32)	Client/SO talking/response time
4	4	(33)	Behavioral data collection
5	5	(34)	Session goals remained in focus

DIAGNOSIS

S	P		
N/A		(35)	Test administration
N/A		(36)	Clinical observation skills
N/A		(37)	Test interpretation and recommendation
N/A		(38)	Professional report writing

ADDITIONAL CLINICAL RESPONSIBILITIES

S	P		
5	5	(39)	Observed clinic rules
5	5	(40)	Prepared for supervisory conferences
4	4	(41)	Contributed alternative procedures
4	4	(42)	Written work was professional
4	4	(43)	Self-supervision of clinical performance

SUMMARY EVALUATION—GRADING

(ADDITIONAL COMMENTS—SEE BACK)

Task	Total S		Total P		# Items		Average	Program Grade or Rating
Planning	25	+	25	/	12	=	4.16	82% B-
Interactions	39	+	39	/	16	=	4.88	97% A
Management	19	+	19	/	8	=	4.75	95% A
Procedures	58	+	58	/	26	=	4.46	89% B+
Diagnosis	—	+	—	/	—	=	—	—
Additional	22	+	22	/	10	=	4.40	88% B+

FINAL GRADE $\dfrac{\text{Total score}}{\text{(\# scores)}}$ = RECOMMENDED GRADE **4.53 = 91% A-**

GOALS FOR DEVELOPMENT:

1. Vary instructional techniques.
2. Increase use of modeling.
3. Use more specific feedback.

Good job working with B.B. + R.G.! thanks.

CBS END OF TERM SELF-SUPERVISION FORM

NAME _K.L.M._ CLINICAL LEVEL* _A_ DATE _5-15-88_ CLIENT _J.C.C._

SUPERVISOR _R.L._ AGENCY _UALR/UAMS_

*Clinical Level: B/eginning: 0–100 HOURS; I/ntermediate: 100–200 HOURS; A/dvanced: 200–300 HOURS; P/rofessional: CFY/BEYOND

NOTE: 1. Rate only *pertinent* behaviors. Use "Key to Clinical Competencies" to rate amount of supervision (S), first column, and quality of performance (P), second column. 5 = Very good; 4 = Good; 3 = Satisfactory; 2 = Less than satisfactory; 1 = Poor.
2. Numbers in ( ) refer to the description of the particular behavior in the "Behavioral Descriptors."
3. SO = significant others.

PLANNING

S P

_3_ _5_ Did you plan reasonable and appropriate semester goals and daily semester objectives? Did you research material for better understanding of the disorder? (1,5)

_4_ _4_ Were you familiar with client's needs so you could effectively plan therapy or a conference? (2,3)

_3_ _4_ Did you select, organize and use goal-oriented materials? Did you plan activities that were interesting and motivating? (4)

_2_ _3_ Did you include SO in planning for therapy? (8)

INTERACTIONS: CLINICAL AND SUPERVISORY

_5_ _5_ Did you build rapport with client/SO that was based on sensitivity, respect, and caring? (9,10)

_5_ _5_ Were you enthusiastic and creative, and did your affect indicate that you enjoyed what you were doing? (11)

_5_ _5_ Did you keep personal factors from interfering with clinical responsibilities? (12)

_4_ _3_ Did you demonstrate initiative, independence, and self-confidence in your clinical management? (13,14)

_5_ _5_ Did you build rapport with your supervisor and appropriately respond to supervision? (15)

_2_ _3_ Did you appropriately inform clients/SO regarding clinical matters? (16)

MANAGEMENT

_4_ _4_ Were lesson plans and progress/diagnostic reports accurate, professional, and turned in on time? Did you keep the files current? (18)

_5_ _4_ Did you create a clinical environment that was conducive to learning or testing? Did you use stimulus control? (19)

_3_ _3_ Did you effectively deal with any behavior problems? Did you use a consistent reward/penalty system? (20)

_3_ _4_ Did you maintain client/SO attention and motivation? Did your client/SO exhibit approach motivation? (21)

PROCEDURES

_4_ _4_ Were your behavioral expectations clear to your client/SO? (22)

_3_ _5_ Was your therapy always focused on goals? Did your goals remain in focus throughout your sessions? (23,34)

_3_ _4_ Were your materials and activities the most efficient/effective means of eliciting goal-directed behavior? (24)

_4_ _4_ Did you use appropriate instructional techniques? (25)

_5_ _5_ Did you discriminate errors from target behaviors, acccurately interpret reponses of SO? (26)

_5_ _5_ Did you demonstrate appropriate pacing of therapy/conference? (27)

_5_ _4_ Did you continuously monitor and adjust to client's/SO's changing needs and performance? (28)

_4_ _4_ Did you use modeling, guidance, and information that was appropriate to the disorder, client, and SO? (29)

_3_ _3_ Did you use a reward and penalty that was appropriate, consistent, verified, etc.?

DIAGNOSIS

_4_ _4_ Did you administer all formal tests accurately and efficiently? (35)

_4_ _4_ Did you demonstrate accurate clinical observation skills? (36)

_4_ _3_ Did you elicit and evaluate all appropriate speech/language/hearing behaviors? Did you accurately interpret test results and make all appropriate recommendations? (37)

ADDITIONAL CLINICAL RESPONSIBILITIES

<u>4</u> <u>4</u>   Were you familiar with the clinic's policies and procedures, and follow the rules and guidelines? Did you take the initiative to fulfill practicum requirements? Was your attire always appropriate for professional activities? (39)

<u>5</u> <u>4</u>   Were you in attendance and on time for all conferences, therapy, and other called meetings? Were you prepared for each conference? Did you actively participate? (40,41)

<u>5</u> <u>4</u>   Did you evaluate your own clinical performance after every session? Did you set goals for your own professional development? Did you accomplish your goals? (43)

CRITIQUE OF OVERALL CLINICAL PERFORMANCE:

I enjoyed my clients this semester but I found the voice and fluency clients the most challenging because I had not had these before. I needed more help applying what I learned in those classes than I expected.

GOALS FOR DEVELOPMENT:

1. Develop strategies for informing SO of clinical progress and including them in therapy.

2. Need more practice in test interpretation. Can I be on another diagnostic team next term?

3. Need to develop more strategies for behavior management. I plan to take the Psych. course in behavior modification next term. I need it!

4. Try to diversify my activities for adult clients. Most of what I had prior to this semester was for children.

I've learned a lot! KSM

Subject Index